Ric Martney
LSU School of
Medicine

PRACTICAL BIOMECHANICS FOR THE ORTHOPEDIC SURGEON

PRACTICAL BIOMECHANICS FOR THE ORTHOPEDIC SURGEON

Eric L. Radin, M.D.
Associate Professor in Orthopedic Surgery Harvard Medical School; Lecturer in Mechanical Engineering, Massachusetts Institute of Technology; Associate, Museum of Comparative Zoology, Harvard University.

Sheldon R. Simon, M.D.
Instructor in Orthopedic Surgery, Harvard Medical School; Lecturer in Mechanical Engineering, Massachusetts Institute of Technology.

Robert M. Rose, Sc.D.
Professor in Materials Sciences and Engineering, Massachusetts Institute of Technology; Lecturer in Orthopedic Surgery, Harvard Medical School.

Igor L. Paul, Sc.D.
Associate Professor in Mechanical Engineering, Massachusetts Institute of Technology; Lecturer in Orthopedic Surgery, Harvard Medical School.

Illustrated by Robin Lefberg

A WILEY MEDICAL PUBLICATION
JOHN WILEY & SONS
New York • Chichester • Brisbane • Toronto

Library of Congress Cataloging in Publication Data:

Main entry under title:

Practical biomechanics for the orthopedic surgeon.

   Includes index.
   1. Orthopedic surgery.   2.   Human mechanics.
3. Spine. 4. Fractures. 5. Joints. 6. Sports—Acci-
dents and injuries. 7. Orthopedic apparatus. I. Radin,
Eric L. [DNLM: 1. Biomechanics. 2. Orthopedics.
WE103.3 P895]
RD732.P7   617′.3   78-11671
ISBN 0-471-02703-0

10 9 8 7 6 5 4 3 2

Preface

This book is based on a post-graduate course on biomechanics for orthopedic surgeons given under the auspices of Harvard Medical School for the past several years. Our emphasis has always been on the clinical applications of biomechanical principles. We have departed, in this book, from the popular practice of teaching biomechanics by developing the basic principles first and subsequently applying them, as is done in engineering education. Since the audience in this case is medical, the basic principles are developed from clinical examples that are familiar to the student. The relevant engineering principles involved in a clinical problem are fully discussed, even if this entails repeating certain principles from one chapter to the next. We feel such repetition is good pedagogy. Likewise, we have not hesitated to sacrifice rigor for the sake of effective teaching. For a fully rigorous exposition of the principles involved, we can only recommend courses in materials science.

We wish to thank all our students who filled out critiques at our courses. This feedback has in large part directed our efforts. We also wish to thank Robin Lefberg, our illustrator, whose genius for clarifying is graphically apparent in the text; Christine Byda, who started typing drafts of this work several years ago and uncomplainingly followed through to the end; and our wives and children whose family lives were chronically disrupted by this effort.

The Authors

Contents

1
Biomechanics of the Spine

1. FUNCTIONAL ANATOMY

The function of the spine is to support the upper torso in various positions, providing sufficient flexibility for trunk movement while at the same time protecting the spinal cord from injury. Activities of daily living require sophisticated trunk motions such as bending, twisting, and carrying loads. These functions must be performed with extreme stability, because spinal dislocation is always disabling and can be catastrophic. Motions of the spine are never frail and "relaxed," but are the result of highly sophisticated bony and soft tissue interactions in concert with active muscle contracture.

The human spine is composed of a series of bone segments connected by discs and ligaments. Flexibility of this rod-like support is achieved by small displacements of its multiple linkages (Fig. 1.1). The advantage of this configuration is that only slight movement of each disc and ligament is necessary for a large,

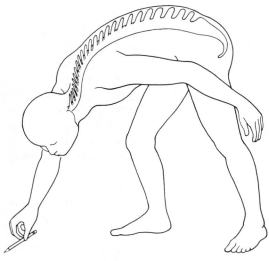

Figure 1.1. High degree of flexibility achieved in the trunk by small displacements of multiple linkages.

overall range of motion. An inherently stable situation is also created by multiple, relatively immobile segments rather than a few highly mobile articulations.

Despite its structural suitability, the spine is prone to mechanical failure. This chapter examines some of these failures and discusses how mechanical factors may influence their occurrence and subsequent treatment. Each type of failure is used to introduce biomechanical concepts of general interest and utility.

2.   COMPRESSION AND COMPRESSION FRACTURES

*Compression** is most simply described as a squeeze. The spine is normally subject to compression due to the weight of the upper body. It is constructed to resist considerable squeezing without crushing. Piled one on top of another, each vertebral body and disc is subjected to the same compressive force. Each unit that is being compressed is deformed by shortening along the direction of compressive force (longitudinal contracture) while expanding laterally (Fig. 1.2). The resistance each has to fracture (*strength*) in this case from crushing, depends on two factors: the geometry (size and shape) of the structure and the material of which it is made.

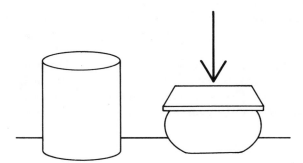

Figure 1.2. When a force is applied to an object to squeeze it, distortion occurs to accommodate this. Note the decrease in overall height and the "barreling" under compressive load.

Suppose two identical vertebral bodies are placed side by side. Are they twice as capable of resisting being crushed as one, that is, are they twice as strong? Intuitively we realize that the strength of each vertebra (in compression) is equal, but now there are two and the same compressive force is distributed over twice the area (Fig. 1.3). Thus each vertebra receives only half the compressive force and is squeezed 50% less than if one vertebral body alone were present. The strength of each vertebral body has not inherently increased because of its own structure but the stress on each has been reduced because the supporting area has doubled. This has effectively halved the load that each segment is subjected to. In order to eliminate the effect of the geometry we can divide the load by the cross-sectional area and obtain the compressive *stress* or force per unit cross-

*Italicized terms are defined in the glossary that follows Chapters 1 through 4.

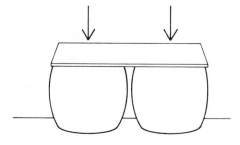

Figure 1.3. If the same amount of force as shown in Fig. 1.2 is distributed over two objects of the same size, each object receives only half the load and is therefore deformed half as much. Consequently, the compressive *stress* on each is one-half what it would be if only one of the two objects received the entire force.

sectional area. Units for stress are the force per given area: newtons per square meter (N/m^2), pounds per square inch (psi), and so on. Thus, in discussing the intrinsic strength of vertebral body material, the mechanical stress present is the relevant quantity.

Suppose we place the same stress on a disc and a vertebral body. What is the resistance of each to being crushed, in other words, how strong is each? Under the same stress, the vertebral body is deformed less than the disc. The bone is stiffer than the disc. Under the same compressive stress the difference in the amounts of deformation produced reflects how much more deformable the disc is than the vertebral body. But it can accurately reflect this only if both were of the same height to begin with. Again, to characterize the material rather than the geometry, the total deformation has to be divided by the overall height. The result is the fractional change in length of material and is called a *strain;* in this case a compressive strain. Strain is usually represented as the percent of the initial length the amount of deformation represents. Ten percent strain means the object has been deformed one tenth of its initial length.

Since vertebral bodies, discs, or any other object are compressed only when squeezed, a strain is produced only when a stress arises. Some relationship between these two quantities should exist. For small strains, the relationship is simple and any given material is characterized by a fixed number which is the ratio of the stress divided by the strain. This number is called the *elastic modulus (Young's modulus)* and is used to relate the susceptibility to deformation of different materials. The higher the elastic modulus, the greater the stress that is needed to produce a given strain (deformation) and the stiffer the material. For example, a vertebral body has a higher elastic modulus than the disc; it is stiffer than the disc and, therefore, under the same compressive force deforms less. Thus if a person's spine is shortened by two centimeters over the course of a day, it is predominantly a loss in height of the discs since they are more easily deformed than the vertebral bodies.

The most common injury to the spine is a compression fracture of the vertebral body (Fig. 1.4). Since the vertebral body is stiffer than the disc, why doesn't the disc (which deforms more than the bone) break first? The answer lies in the fact that the point at which deformation becomes so great that the material loses its integrity and breaks varies from material to material. The stress at which the material fails is called its *ultimate strength.* As stiffness varies from material to material, so does ultimate strength, but the two are not necessarily directly related. The bone in the vertebral body is about 100 times stiffer than the material

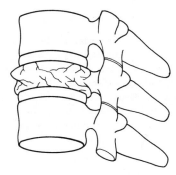

Figure 1.4. Most common injury to the bony spine: compression fracture.

that makes up the disc. Therefore, a given compressive strain (% compression) can be achieved 100 times easier (with 1/100 the amount of compressive stress) in the disc than in the vertebral body. For this reason, under an applied stress below that required to crush bone, disc compressive strain is 100 times as large as the compressive strain in the vertebral bodies, so that almost all of the actual compressive displacement occurs in the disc (Fig. 1.5). Only after the discs have deformed to their maximal strain does the bone begin to crush.

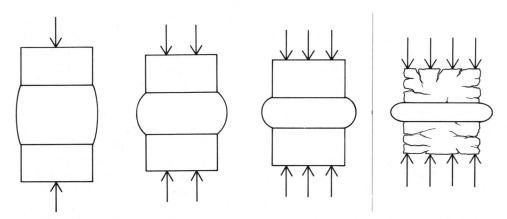

Figure 1.5. Under low to moderate load a vertebral body-disc unit primarily deforms in the structure of the disc. This is because it is not as stiff as the structure of bone. At high loads, however, the breaking strength of bone is lower than that of the disc, and hence ultimate deformation is in the vertebral body.

Bone may fracture owing to abnormal loads that exceed the strength of normal bone or to essentially normal loading patterns when the bone is abnormally weak. Often compression fractures occur in porotic bone under the normal compressive loads of everyday life, because the mechanical character of the bone has changed. Biological materials may change in character depending on alterations in normal physiologic conditions (Wolff's law: disuse atrophy or porosis) or in pathologic conditions (osteomalacia, rickets, idiopathic osteoporosis). These conditions may alter the stiffness of the material (elastic or Young's modulus);

namely, the amount of deformation that occurs with any given stress. Such conditions may also reduce the ultimate strength of the vertebral body; namely, the amount of deformation beyond which the structure is disrupted.

3. MECHANICS OF THE SPINAL COLUMN—NEWTON'S FIRST AND THIRD LAWS

We have considered some properties of the individual components of the spine: the vertebral body and the disc. Let us now consider the basic mechanical properties of the spine itself.

Compressive stress can be produced only if equal and opposite loads are applied to opposite sides of a vertebral body (Fig. 1.6). This is consistent with practical experience. If one applies an unopposed force to one side of an object, that object moves (is pushed) away. In order for an object to remain stationary an equal and opposite force must resist the initial "push." This is in essence *Newton's first law,* which in modified form states that if an object is standing still the sum of the forces acting on it must be zero. Since the vertebral spine does not "fly off into space" or "fall onto the ground," whatever load squeezes it caudal is equally opposed by a cephalad force.

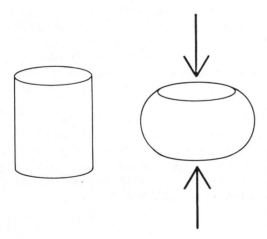

Figure 1.6. If a load is applied to the top of an object, in order for there to be compressive stress on that object, an equal amount of load must be applied to the opposite side, so that the material is squeezed.

If the vertebrae that support a load are stacked, rather than placed side by side, there is no increase in overall compressive strength (Fig. 1.7). The load is transmitted down the column, from one vertebra to the next. Each is loaded as if it were subjected to the entire load. As the load is transferred down the spine, the load on each successive unit is slightly increased by the weight of the vertebrae above it. The cross-sectional area of each vertebral unit increases. One may postulate that this represents an attempt by the body to maintain the same compressive stress at all levels.

In Fig. 1.7B, at the upper vertebra represented, the load is applied to the top. From Newton's first law we recognize that an equal and opposite load must occur at the bottom. The latter is associated with the squeezing together of the two

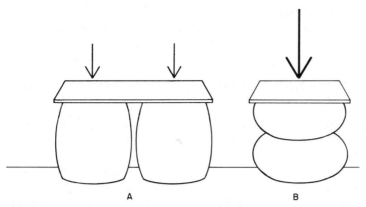

Figure 1.7. If two objects are placed one on top of the other rather than side by side, and the same amount of force is applied to each configuration, stacking provides a smaller area over which the force can be applied. In *B* the cross-sectional area is half that in *A* and hence the compressive forces on the top object are twice as much as on each unit in *A*. In the stack, each unit bears the whole load.

vertebrae. Each vertebra is being compressed. The force at the top of the lower vertebra is equal and opposite to the force at the bottom of the upper vertebra. This is *Newton's third law*: for each action there is an equal and opposite reaction.* The action and reaction are the force exerted by one vertebra on the other and the resulting force on the former. The two laws of Newton (first and third) may be used to deduce the forces on any bone or musculoskeletal element. From the applied forces, the forces on the element and on the remainder of the musculos-keletal system may be determined.

Although the stacking configuration of vertebrae does not change their over-all strength in compression, differences in the dimensional changes occur. Each vertebra and disc in the column is deformed as a relatively independent unit; if we have 10 vertebrae in the stack, each is deformed the same amount under the same circumstances, since the load on each is identical (Fig. 1.8). For the stack of 10, there is an overall diminution of length equal to that of ten vertebrae.

4.   TENSION

It is common in orthopedics to apply skeletal traction in the treatment of cervical fracture-dislocations. A force is applied to the spine in an attempt to restore the individual segments to their original shape and position. It is a force applied in *tension* (Fig. 1.9).

Each vertebral body, disc, and associated ligamentous structures receives this tension as the traction force is opposed by body weight and initially by muscle spasm acting in the opposite direction. If the supine patient is not pulled toward

*The equal and opposite "reaction" is not limited to force but may include movement. We discuss movements of the spinal segments along with scoliosis, lordosis, and spinal fracture-dislocation later in this chapter.

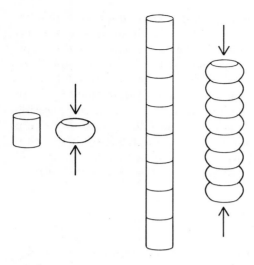

Figure 1.8. Since each unit in a stacked position has the same amount of load applied to it as every other unit, whatever is produced in a single unit is multiplied by the total number of units involved to give the total deformation of the loaded stack.

the head of the bed by the traction, the forces are balanced, according to Newton's first law. No motion occurs and the paravertebral soft tissues are effectively stretched. Under such stretching, discs deform by elongating and narrowing and the paraspinal ligaments are stretched as well. In the area of fracture, ligaments remaining are not restrained by bony contiguity. They deform and stretch the most. Movement of the vertebral bodies is then guided by these soft tissues and the fracture is usually reduced.

All the concepts that apply to compression—stress, strain, and elastic

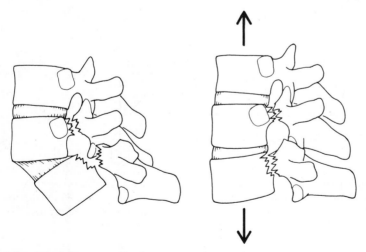

Figure 1.9. In fresh dislocations of the cervical spine, various ligamentous structures as well as bony units are disrupted. The disrupted structures are not as rigid with regard to an applied tensile force. Under such circumstances, greater deformation occurs in these regions than in adjacent regions. For this reason, not uncommonly the fragments can be realigned and reduced by traction.

(Young's) modulus—apply to tensile forces as well. *Tensile stress* is obtained by dividing the load by the cross-sectional area just as with compressive stress. *Tensile strain* is also defined exactly as is compressive strain. The only difference between tension and compression is the direction in which the load is applied to a given body and the subsequent manner in which that body is deformed. In many materials, particularly metals and ceramics, the amount of deformation (strain) per unit force is the same regardless of whether it is in tension or compression. The ratio of stress to strain is the elastic (Young's) modulus in tension or compression. This means that the elastic modulus is the same for tension and compression in most structural materials. However, for soft tissues the elastic modulus is greater for tension than for compression while in bone the reverse is true.

5. SHEAR

If 50 newtons (10 pounds) of cervical traction is applied to a supine patient while in bed, the patient tends to slide toward the head of the bed. Body weight is directed vertically and the traction is horizontal, that is, they are 90° to each other and therefore are not equal and opposite. (Newton's first law explains this.) If a series of rollers were between the patient and the bed, the patient would move and no force would develop in the cervical vertebrae. But if the patient is kept from moving freely, tension develops in his neck. The sheets resist the body's cephalad movement. Such a force applied parallel to a body is a *shear* force (Fig. 1.10).

All the concepts of stress (force per unit cross-sectional area) and strain (% elongation) are equally applicable for shear. Biological materials are weak with regard to shear strength.

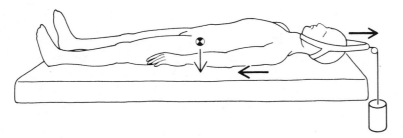

Figure 1.10. In a supine patient the force applied by cervical traction is resisted by a shear force between the patient's body and the bed. The amount of shear force developed depends upon the body weight of the patient. A fat patient in traction is less likely to slide up in bed than a skinny one.

6. VECTORS

Orthopedic surgeons know from experience that the head of the bed must be raised to keep patients who are in strong cervical traction from sliding toward the head of the bed. The reason this works is that, by providing an angle up for the body, the body's weight adds to the shear stress holding the patient onto the sheets (Fig. 1.11). By altering the direction in which the shear force is applied, the vertical force of gravity now contributes to the shear force.

The effectiveness of any force depends upon the direction in which that force is applied. If the shear force remains in a horizontal direction, consider the effect of applying a horizontal force (Fig. 1.12) versus applying a vertical force (Fig. 1.13). Except for indirectly increasing the resistance between the body and the sheets, a vertically applied force has no direct effect. The horizontally applied force acting in the same direction as the shear force contributes all of its magnitude to resisting the traction.

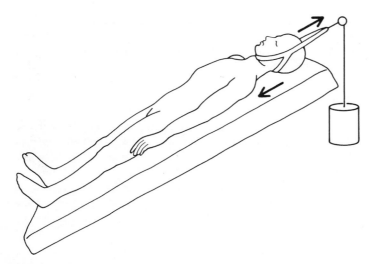

Figure 1.11. By elevating the head of the bed, a component of body weight is in line with that of the shear forces between the body and the sheets of the bed. It therefore contributes to the restraining forces equal and opposite to the traction forces placed on the head by the halter.

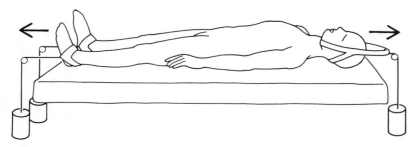

Figure 1.12. An additional force can be applied to counteract the head halter if traction forces are placed on the torso or legs and aligned parallel with the shear forces of the body against the sheets. In the above case, all of the force of the "leg" traction is added to the shear forces of the body against the sheets.

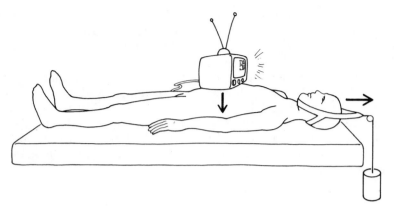

Figure 1.13. Placing a weight on top of the body, perpendicular to the shear force between the sheets and the body, does not contribute any component of force in a direction to help resist the head halter traction. It does contribute by increasing the friction (shear force) between the bed and the sheets.

Now consider some other force directed at some angle between the vertical and horizontal (Fig. 1.14). Whatever component of that force acts in the horizontal direction creates a shear stress in this case. What *component of a force* acts in a particular direction can be most easily determined graphically, as in the bottom of the illustration. The graphic representation of a force or its components is called a force *vector,* such as an arrow with its head showing the direction of the force and the length of the arrow proportional to the magnitude of the force.

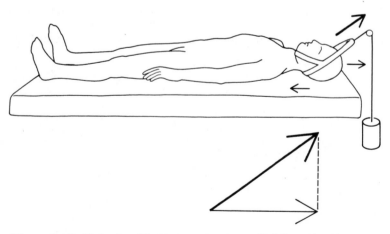

Figure 1.14. If the head halter traction is applied in a direction that is not parallel to the incline of the body against the sheets, only a component of that force in the direction parallel to the body is resisted by the shear forces of the sheets and body.

7. FORCES APPLIED VERSUS STRESSES DEVELOPED

Forward movement of L-5 on S-1 in a patient with spondylolisthesis is produced because of the action of shear forces. The amount of movement is determined by the magnitude of the component of the resultant body weight force in the direction parallel to the vertebral body-disc junction. As the patient leans forward, body weight still acting in a vertical direction produces less compressive force and more shear force at L-5,S-1 (Fig. 1.15).

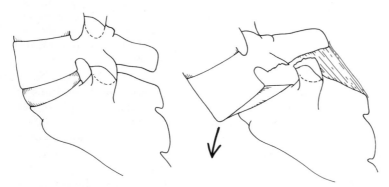

Figure 1.15. When the body is in the upright position, the vertical force of body weight, when aligned over the vertebral body, is practically perpendicular to the vertebral body-disc interface. Under such circumstances, compression between the two units is the major type of stress existing. If, however, the body leans forward, then the vertebral body-disc junction becomes more parallel to the vertical force line of the body weight. In such a circumstance, a substantial component of body weight becomes parallel to the disc-body junction, thus creating shear forces between the two. Under such circumstances, the force creates movement unless an equal and opposite force of the same magnitude develops. This occurs only when the ligaments are strained to the appropriate point.

These increased shear stresses produce movement if an equal and opposite stress is not produced by the disc or ligaments (remember Newton's first law). Such a degree of resistive stress occurs only when the strain of elongation in these tissues reaches certain limits. Up to that point one body slips forward on another. When equilibrium is reached all further movements stop. Hence what appears to be a grade I slip on lying down, can become a grade III spondylolisthesis because of the shear forces created during forward leaning.

What happens if there is no spondylolisthesis? What prevents forward movement? Do shear forces still develop in the disc area? As the body bends forward, if the vertebral body and disc alone were considered, the situation would be the same as that noted above for patients with spondylolisthesis. But normally, articular facets are connected to the vertebral bodies. The geometry of these facets is such that as the body bends forward, the same body weight force acting in the direction that would create shear forces on the vertebral body and disc creates compressive forces at the articular facets (Fig. 1.16).

The magnitude of the forces is the same in both cases, except one is coun-

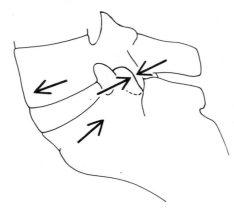

Figure 1.16. Shear forces that develop as a person leans forward are applied to the posterior facet joints. Since they are aligned perpendicular to the direction of the force, the two sides of the joint are squeezed together. In such a case, they are under compression and movement is prevented because the strength of the bone in compression is sufficiently high.

teracted by a shear force, the other by a compressive force. Since the bone in compression is stiffer than the bone and disc in shear, movement is prevented because for the same force the strain developed in compression is small. No movement occurs. The bone takes all the stress. The strain developed in shear in the disc is therefore small. The articular facets act to resist compression and thus save the disc from significantly deforming shear stresses by not allowing any significant strains to develop. In the case of asymmetric L-5,S-1 facets, when facet alignment is altered, the body weight force as the person bends is no longer directed as a compressive force at these facets but as shear (Fig. 1.17). The disc and ligaments are poorly protected by an asymmetric facet joint.

8. BENDING

We have just seen how under the same load parts of a vertebra can sustain different types of stresses owing to structural geometry. The types of stresses

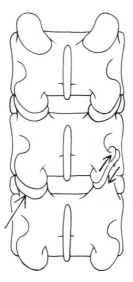

Figure 1.17. Facets normally convert shear at the disc space into compression across the facet joint. If a facet joint is not perpendicular to the intervertebral shear, then instead of acting to compress the joint, a component of the shear acts to make the joint slide. Such a malaligned or "asymmetric" joint cannot bear its share of the compressive stress.

that can be developed in different parts of the disc-vertebral body segment can also differ if the load applied is eccentrically placed. If we return to the L-5,S-1 segment, the examples illustrated above are not quite correct. The load when the person was standing was said to be located directly over the disc and the vertebral body (pure compression); and the load when the person was leaning forward was said to be parallel to the spinal axis and perpendicular to the disc-vertebral body interface (significant shear). In actuality pure compression, tension, and shear are not common in the skeleton, and, owing to the irregular shapes of the body's supporting structures, applied loads tend to rotate or bend the body, as well as squeeze, stretch, or shear it. Such eccentric loading tends to bend the spine (Fig. 1.18).

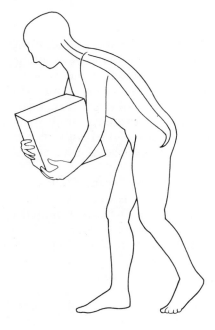

Figure 1.18. When a person picks up an object, the object is not in line with the structures supporting it. Under such circumstances, the person's trunk is not purely squeezed or stretched, but tends to rotate or bend.

Bending involves simultaneous tension and compression stresses at different locations within the same body. When the spine is flexed on the posterior convex side the interspinous ligaments, ligamentum flavum, and posterior longitudinal ligaments are stretched. On the anterior concave side the disc and vertebral body are compressed. Each is deformed and an amount of stress produced is in accord with Young's modulus for bone, disc, and ligament as discussed in Section 2.

Bending has therefore stretched the posterior convex side (made it longer than it originally was) and compressed the anterior concave side (made it shorter than it originally was). In some plane between the concave side and the convex side there is no stretching or compression (ie, no change in length). At this point since length is not changed, there is no strain and hence no stress. More accurately, it is the central plane on which the stresses and strains due to bending equal zero. This plane is referred to as the *neutral plane*.

In a simple bar subjected to pure bending (Fig. 1.19) with a rectangular, round,

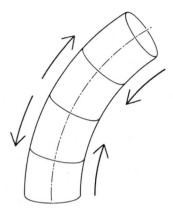

Figure 1.19. When an object is bent, the area on the convex side is stretched and on the concave side is compressed. At some point the decreasing compression changes over in the material to increased stretching. The line or plane up and down the object connecting all those points is called the neutral axis.

or similarly symmetric cross-section, the neutral axis is the central plane of the bar—the plane that cuts the bar in half lengthwise, in the plane of bending. When a column is bent, the fibers on the convex side are stretched and those on the concave side are compressed. From the convex side to the center of the column the fibers are stretched decreasingly; completely unstressed fibers lie on the neutral axis. From that point on the fibers are increasingly compressed. From the center to the concave side the compressive strain (and stress) increases linearly to a maximum at the surface. The linear increase in strain is just a matter of geometry.

Fig. 1.20 shows the stress and strain versus distance from the center line of the bar. The outer surfaces on which the tensile-compressive stresses are maximum are referred to as the *extreme fibers*. Although the spinal column has no symmetric geometry and is certainly not a homogeneous material, these basic concepts of bending apply. As an example, rupture of the anterior longitudinal ligament

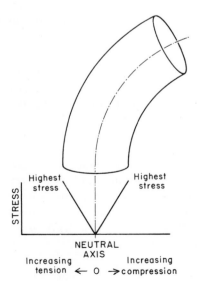

Figure 1.20. When an object is bent, the further away from the neutral axis, the larger the stresses become, since the more the material is either stretched or compressed. On the convex side, the material is stretched and tensile stresses occur; on the concave side, compressive stresses occur.

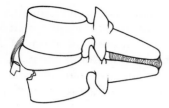

Figure 1.21. Common fracture illustrating bending occurs after forced hyperextension of the cervical spine. A piece of bone is pulled off by the tensile forces created at outermost fibers of bending. Since the bone is weaker under maximum loads than the ligament, the material that breaks under maximum tension is bone rather than ligament.

and bone at C-5 is presumably due to hyperextension in bending. These structures are at the extreme fiber in tension (Fig. 1.21).

Now we return to the stresses present at L-5,S-1. When comparing forward flexion to the upright posture the amount of compressive strain at the disc due to bending may increase. The amount it increases depends on whether the tensile modulus of the ligaments is greater than the compressive modulus of the disc (Fig. 1.22), that is, whether the ligaments are stiffer than the disc. If the ligament is stiffer in tension than the disc is in compression, at a given strain the stresses are higher in the ligament than in the disc. The forward bending load of the body is therefore balanced more by the opposing forces in the ligaments than by those in the disc. The posterior ligamentous structures prevent excessive stresses in the anterior aspects of the disc just as the articular facets usually prevent excessive shear stresses in the disc. The implications of this to the production of pain are interesting since, although the disc is aneuronal, the ligaments and facet joint capsules are well innervated, particularly with stretch receptors.

An interesting implication arises from observing the stress and strains that might be produced in each ligamentous structure when the body bends forward and the ligaments are stretched. If the posterior longitudinal ligament, the ligamentum flavum, and the interspinous ligament all have the same length, cross-sectional area, and modulus of elasticity before bending starts, then the maximum tensile stresses develop in the ligament having the maximum deformation during bending, that is, the interspinous ligament. This ligament is furthest from the neutral axis and is stretched the most in all attitudes of bending. Since we have assumed that the strength and cross-sectional area of all ligaments are the same, and stress and strain are directly related, the ligament that is strained the most has the highest stresses. If, however, the modulus of elasticity for each ligament is different, then the tensile stresses that develop in each ligament are determined not only by the amount of stretch present but also by the strength of each ligament. Depending on the stiffness of each ligament, it

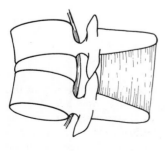

Figure 1.22. If the amount of material or strength of the material on one side of bending is not the same as on the other side, the stiffest material limits the degree of bending that occurs. If, for example, the ligaments on the posterior elements of the spine are stiffer than the disc, the amount of deformation in forward flexion depends more on the geometry of the posterior elements than the disc. In such cases, high compressive stresses are prevented in the disc because of the posterior structures.

is possible that at one particular point of bending, deformation of each ligament, though different, is such as to make the stresses in each ligament the same, that is, the load can be equally shared by all three structures. At other positions of bending, it is possible that the ligament not having the maximum deformation may be under the highest stress. For example, if the ligamentum flavum were stiffer than either the posterior longitudinal or interspinous ligaments, even though the ligamentum flavum is stretched to a length somewhere between the two, the tensile stresses might be the highest in this ligament and it is the one that restricts further movement. A similar situation may arise if the cross-sectional areas of the ligaments differ.

An ingenious mechanism by which the body could provide for sharing the stresses between these three structures would be to have different stiffnesses (moduli of elasticity) and cross-sectional areas in each ligament and at the same time allow each ligament to stretch within a different range of their length. Under this situation their strains are not proportional merely to the distance each ligament is from the center of bending. Such a situation appears to closely resemble what we know to be the case in real life. The posterior longitudinal, ligamentum flavum, and interspinous ligaments all appear to have different resting lengths. It is interesting to reflect on the changes in stress distribution that might arise if with laminectomy any of these tissues is replaced with scar, which might be considered to have a lower stiffness than any of these original ligaments and is stressed the least. Such a situation probably arises with removal of the ligamentum flavum during laminectomy. Under such circumstances since some of the stiffness of the overall structure has been removed and replaced by a much weaker structure, greater deformations may be permissible and significant alterations in the stress distribution result. Hence a degree of instability may arise from laminectomy alone, without disc removal.

Let us return to two other factors that protect the disc from the increased compressive stresses when the body bends forward. The first is the added protection resulting from active contracture of the extensor muscles. With flexion at L-5,S-1, these muscles are active. Since they are eccentrically placed posteriorly, they produce bending in a direction opposite to that produced by body weight (Fig. 1.23). As the body bends forward, the position of these muscles toward the

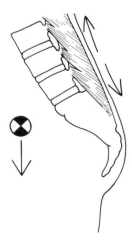

Figure 1.23. Muscle activity at the most posterior aspect of the spinal structure creates a bending moment opposing that of body weight. Contraction of these muscles tends to compress the posterior elements and stretch the anterior elements, and thus nullifies the body weight bending moment. The stresses on the spine created by bending are reduced.

extreme fiber in tension provides them with significant mechanical advantage. If the muscles acted alone, they would create compression in the posterior elements and tension in the anterior elements. Acting in concert with the forward body weight, they neutralize the bending effects of body weight. The posterior muscles act to reduce the tensile stresses in the posterior ligamentous structures and the compressive stresses in the anterior aspect of the spine, protecting the entire structural system from excessive bending stresses. Imagine then the increase in stress and strain created to these structures if the extensor muscles are weak, or if because of denervation they cannot act.

To fully understand the mechanics of the spine in bending let us consider a pressurized fluid within a rigid walled cylinder. The abdominal cavity may be likened to a balloon placed within a tin can. Compression of the balloon from any direction generates pressure that is equal in all directions. This *hydrostatic pressure* can support loads (Fig. 1.24). The lateral walls resist the tendency of the balloon

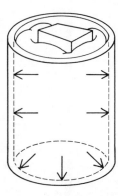

Figure 1.24. When a load is placed on a constrained bag it generates an internal, hydrostatic pressure which can support a load.

to bulge (or bend) outward. The constrained balloon can support the weight at a given height without further deformation. The abdominal cavity, if its walls do not deform (ie, when the abdominal muscles firmly contract), can support some weight of the body above (Fig. 1.25).

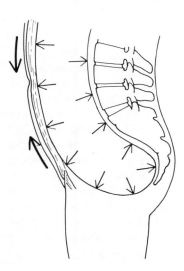

Figure 1.25. The abdominal cavity may be considered a water-filled balloon. It can support some of the weight of the upper body if lateral deformation of it under load can be prevented by containment. Such constraint is provided by strong contraction of abdominal muscles.

In a similar manner the anulus fibrosus acts with the nucleus pulposus to support the compressive load across the intervertebral interspace (Fig. 1.26). When the abdominal cavity acts in the manner shown, the load that the spine must bear is thus decreased. When a person bends or lifts a heavy object, the abdominal muscles contract as in a valsalva maneuver. Imagine then the effects on the load the spine must directly bear with abdominal muscle laxity after stretching from obesity, multiple abdominal procedures, or pregnancies. The effect of a corset as a spinal support is obvious. This explains the compressive strains that develop in the nucleus pulposus if the anulus fibrosus is allowed to bulge or is weakened by a rent or a tear in its structure.

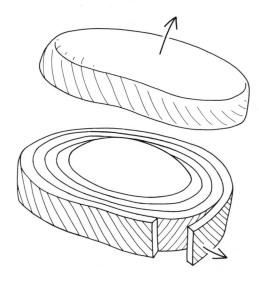

Figure 1.26. The nucleus pulposus and the anulus fibrosus operate in a similar manner to a balloon contained within a can. Hydrostatic pressures are created in the nucleus.

9. STRESS CONCENTRATION—EFFECT OF DISC DEGENERATION AND SPINAL FUSION

An important role of the discs is to evenly distribute the strains in the vertebral bodies and spinal column as a whole. The modulus of elasticity of a disc is much lower than that of a vertebral body and, as mentioned, if a given amount of bending of the back is achieved, it is primarily through the strain produced at the discs. Each disc acts as an articulation and minimizes the bending stresses of the bony portions of the spinal column by allowing the spine to flex at much lower stresses. If a disc degenerates, the space between vertebral bodies narrows and little motion within the segment can occur. What motion does occur is at the posterior elements. Instability results until the deformation creates sufficient stresses to resist further motion. Loss of disc function means greater deformation and greater bending stresses at adjacent discs and vertebrae during a given flexion. A *stress concentration* is thereby produced because of disc degeneration.

A stress concentration is created then whenever rigidity of a section of the vertebral column is increased either by disc degeneration, fusion, or internal fixation devices. The increased stresses so created thus increase the chances of

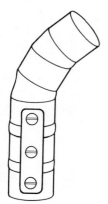

Figure 1.27. If the motion of several vertebral units is restricted by internal fixation or fusion, the same degree of deformation that might occur over five or six segments can occur only over fewer segments. In such circumstances, greater deformation results at each remaining level but, most particularly, the greatest deformation is at the segments just adjacent to the stiffened area, and the stresses in these areas are increased.

spondylolysis (degeneration) or instability in the interspaces at the level of the degenerated disc or above or below a fusion (Fig. 1.27).

The greater the number of rigid segments, the more the remaining segments must deform to achieve the same motion. The more segments fused, the higher the stresses in the adjacent unfused segments. If a plate or a rod is affixed to the spine, the metal is more rigid than the bone. Stresses increase in the surrounding interspaces. Stainless steel or chrome-cobalt alloys, cross-section for cross-section, are 10 times stiffer than bone. If the instrumented spine is strained to achieve the same kind of displacement, much more severe bending stresses in the unreinforced part of the spine exist. Making a section rigid therefore considerably increases stresses in the remaining sections. One can predict traumatic spondylolisthesis just below a Harrington rod fusion for just these reasons (Fig. 1.28).

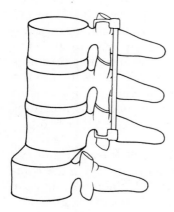

Figure 1.28. Internal fixation with Harrington rods and spinal fusion for scoliosis produces a stress concentration at the level immediately adjacent to it which may lead to a spondylolisthesis.

10. TORSION

We have discussed compression, tension, shear, and bending as they affect the spinal column. One other type of stress has clinical significance for the practicing orthopedist: *torsion*. Torsion stresses in the spine are produced by twisting

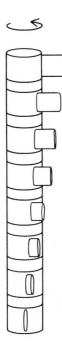

Figure 1.29. Torsion may be defined as a force applied tending to rotate, or twist, a bar about its long axis.

forces—forces applied that tend to rotate the spine about its long axis. When such forces are applied at any vertebral level, that level tends to rotate about the level below (Fig. 1.29).

Motion occurs at the discs as they deform more for given stress (because of lower Young's modulus) than either vertebral body above or below. As torsional forces continue to be applied, the relative motion of one vertebra about the other creates tensile and shear stresses in the anulus fibrosus. Just as in bending the greatest stresses occur in areas furthest from the center of rotation (neutral axis). As they act through the longest lever arms, the facet joints again act to spare the discs from excessive stresses and strains. Unlike bending, rotation produces asymmetric stresses at the joints. With rotation one facet joint closes up and the other opens. Thus compressive and shear stresses are concentrated at one joint while tensile stresses are concentrated in the capsular and ligamentous structures of the contralateral one. This is in contrast to similar stresses created by bending felt in both joints.

Frequently rotatory injuries of the spine are associated with fractures of the facets which act to block excessive rotation. At low levels of the spine the common torsional injury is the fracture dislocation of T-12,L-1: the thoracolumbar junction (Fig. 1.30). Above this level the thoracic spine is relatively stiff. The facets in this region are relatively horizontal and offer little resistance to torsion except through tensile stresses in the capsule and ligaments. Additional resistance to torsional stresses are produced by the rib cage and the costovertebral ligaments which are far away from the neutral axis of torsional rotation. Below this junction the lumbar region gains increased resistance to deformation by the facet joints' progressive vertical orientation. The T-12,L-1 region, being a transi-

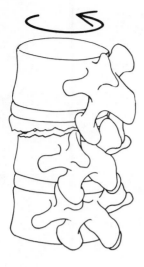

Figure 1.30. Torsion applied to the spine is transmitted from vertebra to vertebra primarily through the facet joints which are compressed on one side and pulled apart on the opposite side. If the torsional force is sufficiently high, bony breakage occurs on the compression side and ligaments rupture on the tensile side.

tional area, has neither the thoracic supplementary protective elements nor the lumbar protective bony geometry, hence torsional deformation and stress are concentrated at the thoracolumbar junction.

11.   LUMBOSACRAL FLEXION EXERCISES AND SPINAL BRACING

From a mechanical point of view repeated flexion of the lumbosacral spine, such as in the Williams Exercise Program, is contraindicated for patients who have spondylosis or spondylolisthesis at L-5,S-1. Such exercises tend to increase the bending stress at this interspace and tend to aggravate whatever structural problems exist. More appropriate treatment for such conditions would be abdominal strengthening exercises done in such a way so as not to flex the lumbosacral junction (Fig. 1.31) and/or abdominal support such as a corset or adequate bracing.

Adequate bracing of the lumbosacral spine must limit both flexion-extension and lateral tilt if it is to completely immobilize that interspace. Braces that do not have trochanteric horns cannot significantly limit lateral tilt (Fig. 1.32). This

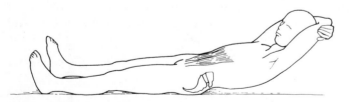

Figure 1.31. Abdominal strengthening exercises should be done in the recumbent position with the lumbosacral spine splinted by the floor or mat. In this position the forces effected by body weight do not act to counter abdominal contraction nor create bending moments in the lumbosacral spine.

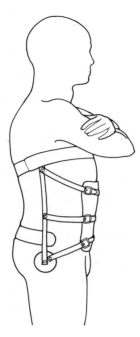

Figure 1.32. The trochanteric pad of a lumbar brace with rigid sides prevents lateral bending.

probably explains the unreliable results chairback braces provide in the treatment of L-5,S-1 disease when lateral tilt causes symptoms. The Norton-Brown brace which provides trochanteric horns would appear to be more effective for the treatment of these conditions. It is also important if flexible pelvic obliquity exists secondary to a leg length discrepancy that the pelvis be balanced with a heel lift or other methods. Pelvic obliquity creates a bending component laterally which puts increased compressive stress across one facet and increased tensile stress across the capsule and ligaments on the opposite side. This necessitates an increased force from the paraspinal muscles on the tension side sufficient to neutralize this bending stress and can be associated with symptoms.

Fixed pelvic obliquities are most commonly associated with scoliosis. This scoliosis often balances the spine above the pelvis. In such circumstances a lift under the shoe may only aggravate the symptoms. A heel lift does not alter a fixed pelvic obliquity. If pelvic obliquity is fixed and a fusion of the scoliosis is performed, the lift only unbalances the trunk and creates a bending moment. In such cases strong consideration should be given to inclusion of the lumbosacral junction in the fusion to both maintain the spine centrally over the sacrum and prevent late degenerative changes at L-5,S-1 below the fusion because of the high stress concentrations from bending stresses which arise.

12.   SPONDYLOLISTHESIS AS A FATIGUE FRACTURE

We have described failures of the spine under various conditions, when the load is too high for the normal structural material to withstand it or the structure's material properties have weakened enabling normal forces to cause failure. Can structures fail under normal forces on normal strength structures?

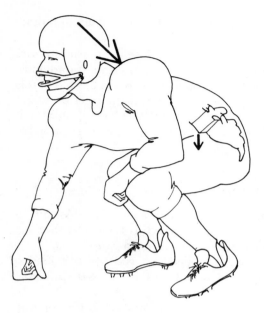

Figure 1.33. Movement of a player from a crouched position would elicit a lordotic type of bending in the lumbar spine. Additionally if the subject is struck in the shoulder or chest region, a significant extension bending moment is created. Repetitive reversals in flexion-extension under such circumstances may cause failure in the area of the pars.

Over the past several years it has become apparent that there is a form of spondylolisthesis that is a slowly developing fracture of the pars interarticularis, most common in adolescents who perform in contact sports and in gymnastics. The mechanism of injury is thought to be impact loading while the L5, S-1 interspace is repetitively flexed and extended (Fig. 1.33). This has to be done on a repetitive basis because the pars interarticularis, unless it has some congenital anomalies, can probably withstand the stress induced by a single normal impact. It is thought that with repetitive, frequent loads the bending stresses eventually produce a small crack. This initially occurs on the tensile (posterior) side of the pars and propagates slowly with each repetitive insult until it works its way completely across the bone (Fig. 1.34).

This fracture occurs much in the same way one breaks a paper clip by bending it repeatedly back and forth. This is known as fatiguing and the subsequent result

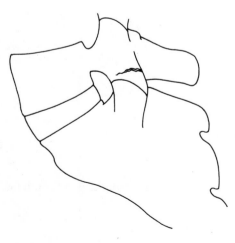

Figure 1.34. In the pars, a fatigue fracture may occur from tensile stresses attempting to separate the bone. Once a crack is started, each flexion and extension further opens this crack, leading to eventual failure.

is a *fatigue fracture,* a ubiquitous engineering problem. More is said about fatigue failure in Chapters 2 and 3.

Such fatigue fractures appear at the pars probably because the tensile stresses in this area of the bone are the greatest. Thus in considering this spondylolisthesis as a fatigue fracture, it implies that if the adolescent who is subjected to this sort of impulse loading avoids such repetitive bending stresses the fracture might heal, if it is still in the incomplete stage. However, once the pars has ruptured, it is relatively unstable and conservative measures that bring about healing in a stable fracture usually do not work.

13.   RESISTANCE OF THE SPINE TO BENDING

We have seen that the spine can be roughly considered as a long, flexible rod. In bending, a rod can be deformed by vertical forces, which is known as *buckling.* The vertical force that begins to produce buckling is called a *critical load.*

In Fig. 1.35 various constraints have been applied to a rod which is loaded vertically and is attached to a base. If no restraint to lateral bending is applied at the top, a minimal load is necessary for buckling and a C-curve results (Fig. 1.35A). If lateral motion of the ends of the rod are restrained, but the top and bottom are allowed to rotate, the force necessary to buckle the rod is increased by a factor of 4 (Fig. 1.35B). Restraints that prevent lateral deviation but allow rotation at the top further double the critical load (Fig. 1.35C). This corresponds to the human situation where lateral deviation is restrained but the upper end of the spine can bend freely while the lower end is fixed through the sacrum to the pelvis. As compared with the unsupported model shown in Fig. 1.35A, this configuration requires eight times the load to buckle. The critical load can be maximized by creating a situation where both lateral deviation and bending at the top and bottom are prevented (Fig. 1.35D).

The human spine is already naturally bent in the sagittal or lateral plane (postural kyphosis and lordosis) (Fig. 1.36). The occurrence of scoliosis (bending

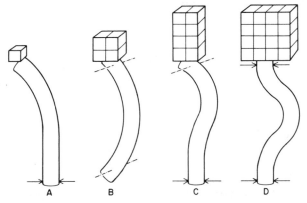

Figure 1.35. The amount of load a column supports without buckling depends on how the column is restrained.

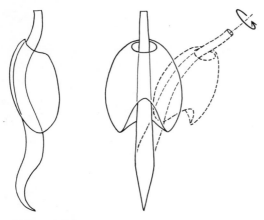

Figure 1.36. The normal spine has a thoracic kyphosis and a lumbar lordosis. The superimposition of a lateral curvature (scoliosis) on this configuration results in an obligatory axial rotation of the spinal column as well.

in the frontal plane) necessitates spinal rotation. This is true because one cannot bend a flexible rod in two planes perpendicular to each other without rotating the rod. The most flexible area of the spine in rotation has been shown to be around T-7. The lumbar facets, because of their more vertical orientation, tend to limit rotation more than do the thoracic facets. It is therefore predictable that the greatest rotatory deformities in a scoliosis occur in the thoracic region.

As pointed out, the flexibility of the spine results to a great extent from the intervertebral discs which allow bending, rotation, and a limited amount of tilt and sideways slip of the vertebrae. Movement beyond these limits requires interruption of the disc and its associated ligaments. The discs contribute not only much of the flexibility of the spinal column but also a major restraint to spinal motion. The resistance of the spinal column, the vertebrae, discs, and ligaments to buckling is small. It requires only about 20 newtons (four pounds) to buckle a thoracolumbar spine that has been dissected out of an adult human cadaver.

However, the critical load that buckles the adult cadaver human spine with ribs and sacrum still attached has been calculated to be about 350 newtons (70 pounds) of force. Interestingly, this is the average combined weight of the upper torso, head, and arms of a normal adult. Stability of the spine against buckling in vivo must obviously involve factors additional to the intrinsic anatomic structures. These extrinsic stabilizing factors are the forces exerted by the trunk muscles. In most cases in a normal spine, symmetric contraction of these muscles prevents buckling but when the spine is rotated and laterally bent, these muscles located lateral to the midline can act as further deforming forces (Fig. 1.37).

Clearly, once an imbalance occurs, the now misaligned muscular forces, or the absence of muscular forces as in paralytic situations, added to the forces produced by the body mass cause the curve to progress further. If this occurs in a growing child, accommodation to the abnormal stress causes uneven epiphyseal growth, vertebral wedging, and permanent bone curvature. Even

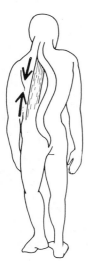

Figure 1.37. In a patient with scoliosis, muscles contracting on the concave side in normal daily activities can cause accentuation of the curve. Muscles on the opposite side may tend to neutralize the curve and attempt to unbend it, but are usually at a mechanical disadvantage.

after growth has ceased the abnormal muscular forces acting on a scoliotic spine in adulthood, through the process of soft tissue remodeling, can cause further progression of curves in a slow but sometimes symptomatically significant fashion.

The mechanical factors that induce scoliotic deformities would therefore be expected to be most effective in the upright posture (Fig. 1.38).

14.   MECHANICS OF STRAIGHTENING A CURVED SPINE

The principle of straightening a curved spine is to unbend it. Consider what sorts of forces are needed to unbend a simple C-curve. It can be straightened by either placing the spine in traction or by pushing laterally on the apex of the

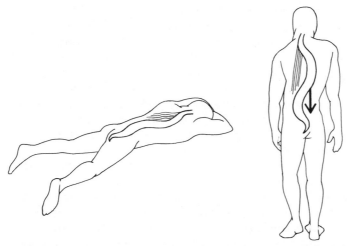

Figure 1.38. Forces to correct scoliosis would be most effective when resistance is minimal. This would occur in the recumbent position, since when the subject is upright, body weight produces bending moments that tend to aggravate the scoliosis.

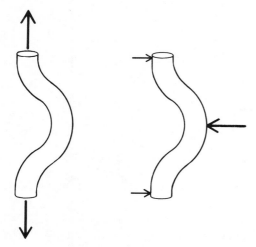

Figure 1.39. To be effective, both traction and pushing on a curved spine to straighten it require equal and opposite forces.

curve. The corrective force must be opposed by equal and opposite forces (Fig. 1.39).

Thus to straighten the spine you must either push or pull against some resistance. Any unopposed force, either a pull at one end of the curve or a push at the apex of the curve, just accelerates the spine and does not straighten it. Remember Newton's first law! Equal and opposite forces must be applied in such a way that the ends of the curve are free to move away from each other as straightening progresses (Fig. 1.40); otherwise only the pattern of curvature may be changed rather than straightening the spine.

In order to straighten a scoliosis curve, forces must act at some distance away from the apex of the curve (Fig. 1.41). The perpendicular distance from the line of application of the force to the apex of the curve is defined as the lever arm or *moment arm* of the force. The longer the lever arm the greater the counter-bending produced. The effectiveness of this counter-bending is determined by multiplying the force by the length of the lever arm. The product of this multiplication is defined as the moment of the force or the *bending moment*.

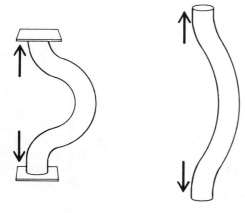

Figure 1.40. If forces are applied to a curve but movement is prevented, all attempts at correction are futile. Movement must be allowed.

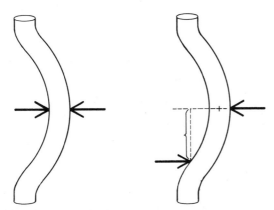

Figure 1.41. Equal and opposite forces applied at the same level on a curve have no rotatory (straightening) effect. For straightening (unbending) to occur the equal and opposite forces have to be applied a distance apart. The magnitude of the (un)bending moment applied depends on the distance of these forces from the center of curvature.

Therefore, bending moments are created either by pulling on the ends of the spine (Fig. 1.43) or pushing in separate places along the spine (Fig. 1.42). Consider these two methods in relatively mild curves. Horizontally applied forces create significant bending moments as their lever arms are relatively large (Fig. 1.42). Traction forces would have to be very large to be effective because the lever arm they work through is relatively small (Fig. 1.43).

In severe curves, traction forces are efficient as they have significantly greater lever arms (Fig. 1.44). Horizontally applied forces are at a mechanical disadvantage (Fig. 1.45), or at least a lesser advantage.

Besides the magnitude of the applied forces, their point of application, and the lever arms through which they function, one other determinant of the effectiveness of a force in creating a relevant bending moment is the direction in which the force is applied. Compare a horizontally applied counter-force to one of similar magnitude and point of application which is skewed from the horizontal (Fig. 1.46). Only the horizontal component of the force helps to

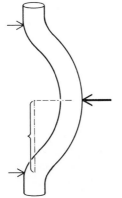

Figure 1.42. The force on the right-hand side of the curve is equal and opposite to the two forces on the left-hand side. No lateral motion occurs. Since the forces are equal and opposite but are not in the same line, that is, spaced a distance apart, the two tend to rotate the top part of the curve clockwise, and the bottom two tend to rotate the bottom part of the curve counterclockwise, thereby straightening the curve.

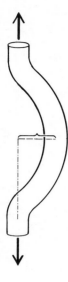

Figure 1.43. Another configuration producing the same result as in Fig. 1.42. Here both forces are off-center; therefore, the top force produces a clockwise bending moment on the top part of the curve, and the bottom force produces counterclockwise bending on the bottom part of the curve. Since the two forces are equal and opposite, the structure does not move up or down but merely straightens.

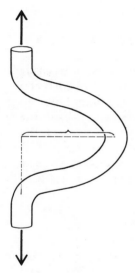

Figure 1.44. In comparison to Fig. 1.43 the same forces applied on a severe curve have a greater tendency to unbend the curve, since the moment arm of each force from the center of rotation is large.

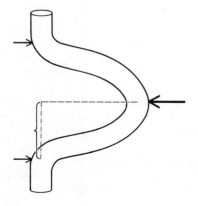

Figure 1.45. If forces of similar magnitudes as in Fig. 1.44 are applied in opposite directions, there is less of a tendency for the curve to be straightened, since, although the magnitude of the forces is about the same, the moment arm of each from the center is less.

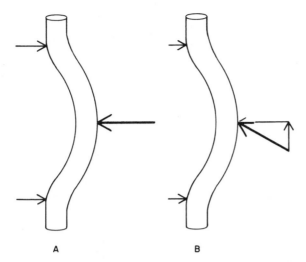

A   B

Figure 1.46. If a force is applied at an angle (as in *B*), only the lateral component of the force acts through a moment arm and contributes to the bending moment.

straighten the curve. The vertical component of the pushing force has absolutely no beneficial effect in this case.

The component of a force that acts in a particular direction can be most easily determined graphically.* When lateral and traction forces combine to correct a curve, both vertical and horizontal forces act at the ends of the spine. One can add the moments of the components that go to make up the *resultant force* in the appropriate directions. The resultant bending moment acting on the spine is the sum of the bending moments contributed by each component of the forces acting in a meaningful fashion on the spine (Fig. 1.47). The *components of a force* which act in a particular direction can be determined graphically (Fig. 1.48).

15.   TRACTION, CASTS, AND BRACES

Traction, casts, and braces either pull or push on the spine and act to correct scoliosis by creating bending moments. The spine can be pulled by skeletal halo-femoral or halo-pelvic traction (Fig. 1.49). Theoretically traction is effective in severe curves if, of course, they are flexible. However, many such curves are stiff and inflexible and the substantial traction forces necessary to overcome them cannot be generated because of the limitations of the holding power of the pins in the bone or the amount of traction the ligaments and discs in the flexible noncurved areas can resist. As a result, combinations of soft tissue releases and skeletal traction make more mechanical sense in severe curves.

Another method of straightening a scoliotic spine is to apply a bending moment to the curve with a turnbuckle jacket (Fig. 1.50). In this technique, a body

---

*Our intuitive isolation of the spine to study the effect of the forces acting upon it is valid from an engineering standpoint as long as we consider all the forces and counterforces at work on this isolated structure. The creation of such an isolated static equilibrium is referred to as *free body analysis*.

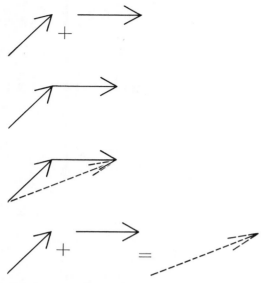

Figure 1.47. When several forces acting on the same body are directed at different angles, the magnitude and direction of the total resulting force acting on that body may be obtained by placing each force head to tail against the other ones, maintaining its direction and representing its magnitude by the length of the line. The resultant force is the line connecting the tail of the first force to the head of the last force.

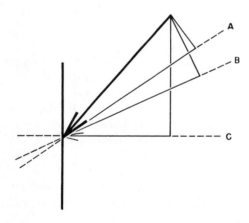

Figure 1.48. A given force has a component in any particular direction (A,B,C) by drawing a right triangle. The base of that triangle then gives the magnitude and direction of that component.

cast is applied with both ends of the spine fixed in the plaster. Hinges are plastered directly over the apex of the curve, and the cast cut so that the top and bottom of the cast can be spread using a turnbuckle. This essentially applies counterbending to the spine with relatively large moment arms. This method is biomechanically very effective. It is limited only by tissue tolerance to the bending moments applied.

A more recent modification of this technique, the localizer jacket, is an attempt to improve on the turnbuckle jacket by applying a body cast while the spine is in traction and adding lateral pressure to the curve through the pusher pads (Fig.

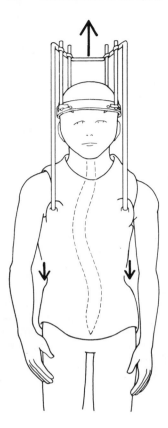

Figure 1.49. Halo-femoral or halo-pelvic traction by fixation to the skull and bony pelvis or femurs. Traction then produces equal and opposite tensile forces which tend to unbend the spine.

1.51). This combination is a mechanically advantageous method of correcting both the severe curve (traction) and the curve as it becomes milder (lateral pressure). As correction is obtained new casts can be applied serially.

This method has been further modified for more practical use by the Milwaukee brace. This device combines traction and pushing forces in such a way that they can be adjusted as the curve corrects as the patient grows (Fig. 1.52). The traction from the Milwaukee brace is mostly achieved by the patient's attempts to stretch out of the brace with his own muscular activity. The brace prevents both lateral deviation and bending, establishing the constraints requiring the greatest critical load to buckle the spine (see Fig. 1.35D). This mechanical situation acts to limit the progression of the scoliosis as gravity and other deforming forces have to be maximal in order to buckle the spine. Lying down obviates these deforming forces and allows the brace to be most effective. Thus, one of the most effective situations for correction exists if the patient wears the Milwaukee brace in bed.

If the extrinsic stabilizing factors (muscular contractions) are absent, minimal forces can buckle the spine and the brace cannot prevent this. This is because the corrective forces that would be required are not tolerated. In a reverse sense the motor strength in patients with scoliosis secondary to spasticity is also usually too great for a Milwaukee brace to overcome. If the extrinsic stabilizing factors are not functioning, progression of the curve within the brace is likely. The use of the

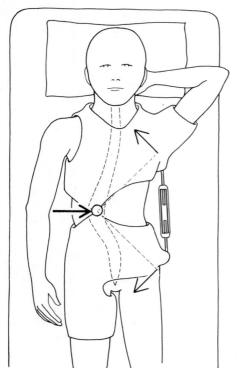

Figure 1.50. A turnbuckle jacket produces equal and opposite forces which, because they are placed off center and have significant moment arms, can unbend a scoliotic curve.

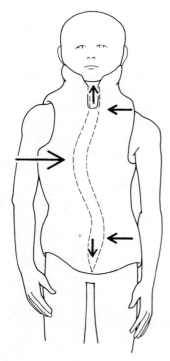

Figure 1.51. A localizer jacket combines tensile traction through the head and pelvis with lateral forces to create bending moments from different directions.

33

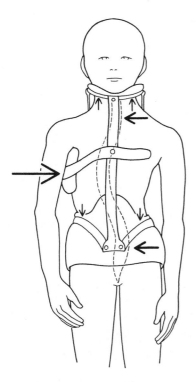

Figure 1.52. A Milwaukee brace has the potential to produce the same type of forces in the same manner as does a localizer jacket. Because the forces are applied at specific points, high pressure may limit the amount of force that can be generated. By the body reacting by "withdrawal" from these contact forces, a similar effect to unbend the spine may occur from muscle activity.

Milwaukee brace would then not be expected to be as effective in the treatment of paralytic curves or in any situation when the patient cannot actively stretch out of the brace and/or the internal forces are high. Such curves should be more responsive to casting or jackets, which act by external containment, as a bucket around the spine creating conditions of maximum constraint to lateral bending and free rotation (Fig. 1.53).

The Milwaukee brace is most effective if the curve is small and the rib pad is arranged almost perpendicular to the spine. The force of the thoracic pad is transferred to the vertebral spine through the ribs as they attach to the vertebral body and transverse processes. Apically placed thoracic pads perpendicular to the long axis of the spine and opposing forces positioned laterally at the pelvis and neck act through long lever arms and create significant moments with relatively small forces.

If the curve is large, the force created by the pad and neck and pelvic supports tends to become more and more parallel to the axis of the curve and less and less corrective. Furthermore, such patients usually have a severe rib deformity. The pad would have to be applied in a more vertical direction because horizontal application would only push the ribs in (Fig. 1.54).

Thus in curves of more than about 60° the Milwaukee brace is not an effective method of treatment. The components of forces and the moment arms acting in a corrective fashion in such a curve are small. The total force applied to create any sort of meaningful bending moment would have to be large. An attempt to use pads to exert force of this magnitude usually causes skin breakdown.

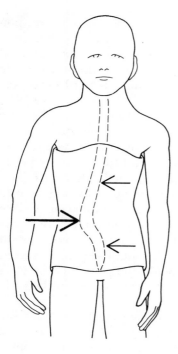

Figure 1.53. A body jacket, which entirely contains an area of the body, prevents bending forces created by the patient's weight from further deforming the spine.

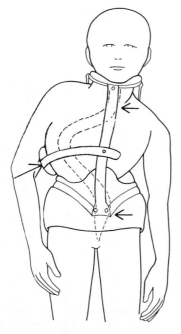

Figure 1.54. The greater the degree of scoliotic curvature, the more parallel the ribs are aligned with a vertical axis. If a pressure pad is to transmit force to the spine through these ribs, the force applied through the pad must become more vertical. If it does not, it would only squeeze the ribs in toward the center of the body. With greater degrees of scoliosis, a limit to the verticality of the applied force is reached, since in the ultimate position (vertical) no force could be transmitted to the ribs since such a force applied externally would merely push the skin upward.

35

In curves of 30° to 60° the success of the Milwaukee brace may depend upon the degree of spinal rotation. Milwaukee braces tend to have maximal therapeutic effect in idiopathic curves of 30° to 60° that do not have a significant rotational component. Rotation in a scoliotic spine is not necessarily proportional to the severity of the lateral bend. When rotation is great, pushing on the ribs probably only increases the rotational deformity.

Just as the Milwaukee brace can be effective in scoliotic curves below 60° its use can be extended to correct kyphosis. Here, in order to unbend the curve, forces must be applied anteriorly and posteriorly, ideally where pressure can be applied directly over the ends and apex of the curves. To unbend the spine the pelvic girdle can apply a force from its anterior surface and a pad in the thoracic region over the sternum can also easily be used. To insure correction and that the entire spine is not just moved posteriorly, a force acting from the posterior surface directed anteriorly is needed. Such a force can be provided directly over the spinous processes with a pad at the apex of the curve. Such three-point fixation applied with sufficient force can achieve the desired result. The forces exerted by the pads have not to date been measured although it appears that they act much in the same way as in scoliosis; they may more actively correct by the body applying the forces themselves (Fig. 1.55).

At the least, it appears that the forces exerted by the pads rigidly maintain the three points at which they are applied and motion initiated by muscle activity and trunk movement produces a relative unbending of the spine about these points. Such activity and motion can be assisted if the weight of the trunk above the apex of the curve can produce a bending force by the shoulder girdle in a direction to correct the kyphosis. Fixation of the pelvis anteriorly, apex of the curve

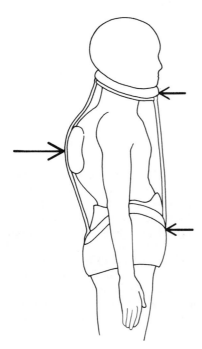

Figure 1.55. A Milwaukee brace can apply forces in the sagittal rather than frontal plane and thus assists in correcting a kyphotic deformity.

posteriorly, and the upper sternum anteriorly hold the trunk in this position and body weight corrects bending forces when the patient is upright.

16. INTERNAL FIXATION DEVICES

In some cases of scoliosis, external casts and braces do not satisfactorily correct the curve. Surgical correction and internal fixation are indicated. Correction is achieved by the same principles as with braces and casts, namely by applying proper bending moments. Harrington instrumentation, an example of this, is a method of straightening the scoliotic spine by implanting parallel compression and distraction rods, which are hooked onto the posterior elements of the spine (Fig. 1.56).

The distraction rods do most of the correction in Harrington instrumentation, much as in halo-pelvic traction or turnbuckle casts. As one starts to apply tension with a Harrington distraction rod the curve begins to straighten out relatively easily. As distraction continues, the more the curve is straightened out the more difficult further correction becomes. At first the distraction force has a large component perpendicular to the bent spinal axis and acts through a relatively long lever arm in relation to the apex of the curve (Fig. 1.57). Such a force therefore effects a favorable counter-bending moment. As the spine straightens,

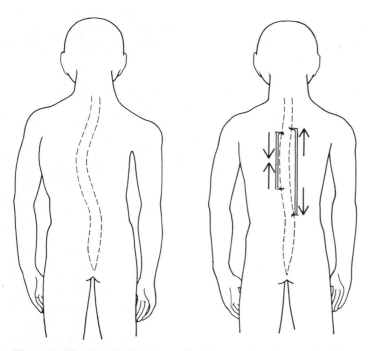

Figure 1.56. Tensile forces applied in equal and opposite directions to the concave side, and compression forces applied to the convex side of the curve, create bending moments which can straighten a scoliotic curve.

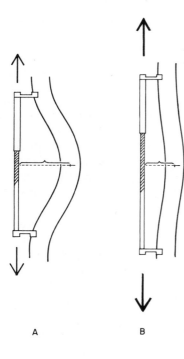

A   B

Figure 1.57. *A,* if tensile forces are applied to the concave side of a curve, small forces are needed if the curve is large, since the bending moment arm is also large. *B,* The straighter the curve becomes, the smaller the bending moment arm. If the same bending moments are to be created, higher tensile forces are needed.

the distraction force tends to become parallel to the spine and its lever arm is progressively reduced. Greater force is necessary to achieve the same bending moment. Correction ceases when the corrective force equals that of the strength of the ligaments and bone.

In both theory and practice, the Harrington compression rod is less effective than the distraction rod. Compression rods are effective only in curves less than about 50°. In curves greater than that most of the force derived from the compression hook is parallel to the axis of the spine and acts only through a short lever arm; hence, not much corrective bending moment is created (Fig. 1.58). Furthermore, in curves of more than about 50° the transverse processes of vertebrae are usually so rotated that the compression rod hooked onto these lies

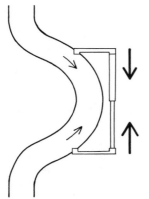

Figure 1.58. If compression forces are applied to the convex side of the curve, the bending moment created is not very large because the moment arm is small. Large compressive forces would therefore be needed and this is limited by the strength of the bone to which the hooks are applied.

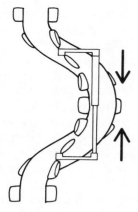

Figure 1.59. In scoliotic curves greater than 50° the transverse processes are rotated to such a degree that they are on the concave side of the curve. If compression hooks were applied to these regions, a bending moment would be created which would increase the curvature.

not on the concave side but actually on the convex side (Fig. 1.59). In such a configuration, attempts at compression actually bend the curve even more. In addition, these transverse processes are pointed more posteriorly than laterally and compression tends to create (or aggravate pre-existing) lordosis (Fig. 1.60).

The strength of the bony attachments into which the hooks of the rods are inserted limit the force that can be applied in either tension or compression. The distraction rod hooks are preferentially placed under the lamina, and, if left intact and not notched, are relatively strong. The compression rod hooks, on the other hand, are put around the transverse processes, which are relatively weak and break if much load is applied to them.

It is important to insure that the instrumented spine is balanced over the sacrum. The lowest hook of the distraction rod should be vertically over the

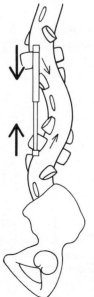

Figure 1.60. The transverse processes in a severely scoliotic curve on the convex side are rotated posteriorly. If lordosis exists the bending moments created by a compression rod increase the lordosis.

sacrum to prevent the center of gravity of any overlying residual scoliotic curve from creating bending moments over the sacrum. This would create another curve between the lower end of the rod and the sacrum (Fig. 1.61).

In the treatment of double curves it is mechanically sounder to use one rod in a dollar sign ($) fashion rather than two separate rods. Each curve has its own degree of flexibility and the chance of straightening the curves equally is unlikely, so that to thus balance the spine as a whole is more likely with one rod than with two. It is mechanically wiser to accept some limitation in correction and end up with a balanced, stable spine. Furthermore, if two rods are used and they do not overlap this creates a gap between two solid areas that acts as an area of stress concentration and high strains result. The chance of fusion in this inter-rod area is reduced.

Harrington rods applied posteriorly can correct lordotic deformities associated with scoliosis but, of course, are less effective in correcting associated kyphotic deformities. Since rods would have to be bent, the component of force acting to correct the curve is reduced. Also application of corrective forces at the ends of the curve, as with Harrington rods, is not mechanically advantageous in short, sharp curves that tend to be rigid in their central portion. It is anatomically impossible to put in Harrington rods if the posterior elements are absent or weak. In such cases another approach is needed.

Dwyer has developed an internal fixation device that can be applied to the anterior aspect of the vertebrae. The spine is approached anteriorly and the intervertebral discs are excised. Removing these discs allows considerable correction as it essentially removes wedges from the concave side of the curve and thus eliminates part of the spine contributing significantly to its rigidity. After the discs are removed, the spine is extremely flexible and can be straightened manually. A cable is then applied with staples and screws to the anterior-lateral aspect of the vertebral body. The cable holds the correction achieved by the surgical excision of discs (Fig. 1.62) (and bone if necessary); it does not function as a corrective force.

This technique allows the individual correction of one vertebral body on its neighbors as the cable is crimped from interspace to interspace. The Dwyer

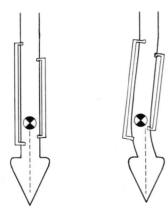

Figure 1.61. If in correcting a scoliotic curvature the final position achieved is centered off the pelvis, a bending moment is created proportional to the weight above the pelvis times the amount off the midline the center of gravity is (moment arm).

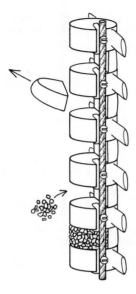

Figure 1.62. If scoliosis is corrected by the anterior approach, removal of the discs takes away a considerable amount of the internal structure that resists unbending the curve. Little external force is therefore necessary to straighten the spine. The Dwyer apparatus can then be used until fusion occurs to prevent body weight and muscle activity from creating bending stresses that might redeform the curve.

apparatus, therefore, does not work on the same principles as the methods of treatment outlined above, by applying a force to unbend a curve. Rather, using the Dwyer method, the surgeon corrects a curve by excising wedges anteriorly, manually straightening out the spine, and then applying a band to resist bending on the tensile side of the corrected curve which prevents the deformity from recurring. If an attempt is made to use the Dwyer apparatus to correct the deformity (by using it to apply bending moments) rather than just to hold the correction, one risks either pullout of the fixation of the cable from the bone due to generation of excessive force or tensile fatigue of the cable from excessive repetitive tensile stress.

GLOSSARY

Bending   Induction of curvature in the long axis of an object by the application of an eccentric force or bending moment.

Bending moment (moment of a force)   Measure of the bending intensity created by a force (obtained by multiplying a force by its lever arm).

Buckling   Bending produced by vertical forces along the long axis of an object.

Component of a force   Portion of a force acting in a particular direction or directions.

Components of force   Breakdown of a force in different directions. The vector sum of all force components is just equal to the original force. Thus deformation and reaction to force components are the same as to the original force.

Compression   Application of force tending to squeeze or crush an object.

Critical load   Vertical force that begins to produce buckling.

Elastic (Young's) modulus   Measure of relative stiffness. It is determined by dividing the stress (newtons/m^2) by the strain (%) and therefore has the same units as the stress. May also be thought of as the proportionality constant relating a material's stress and strain behavior.

Extreme fibers   Outermost fibers on the convex and concave sides of a bent object.

Fatigue fracture   Structural failure caused by repetitive tensile stresses which, although below the ultimate strength, cause a slowly propagating crack to cross the material.

Free body analysis   Method of determining forces acting on a body by isolating that body and assuring it is in static equilibrium.

Hydrostatic pressure   Stress produced by forces acting equally in all directions.

Moment arm   Shortest distance between the line of application of a force and the point around which the moment of the force is being taken.

Neutral axis   Plane in a bent object at which zero stresses and strains occur (usually the center).

Newton's first law   If the sum of the forces on an object is zero the object does not move.

Newton's third law   For each force there is an equal and opposite force.

Resultant force   Sum of force components.

Shear   Force applied parallel to an object's surface (eg, rubbing force). Shearing forces can also exist deep within the material itself.

Static equilibrium   State at which Newton's first law is satisfied.

Strain   Amount of deformation (% elongation) compared to original dimension.

Strength   Maximum resistance to stress before failure.

Stress   Force per unit of area.

Stress concentration   Point of significantly increased stress.

Tension   Application of force tending to elongate an object (a pull).

Torsion   Forces applied tending to rotate an object about its long axis (a twist).

Ultimate strength   Stress at which material ruptures.

Vector   Graphic representation of a force as an arrow. The direction of the arrow is the line of action of the force; the length of the arrow is proportional to the magnitude of the force.

2
Mechanics of Fracture and Fracture Fixation

1. MECHANICS OF FRACTURE

In general when a bone is subjected to a steady load two competing processes occur:

1. *plastic or viscous flow,* in which planes of atoms or molecules slide over each other like a deck of cards: such deformation is caused exclusively by *shear stress.*
2. *fracture,* in which a crack grows from microscopic to large size (sometimes rapidly!). For steady loads, fracture in strong, hard materials such as bone is caused by *tensile stress.*

Fracture is common in the long bones but the origins of the necessary tensile stresses are not clear. For instance, to cause tensile stresses by putting the skeleton in traction would generally result in joint dislocation. Also, muscular contractions always resist such tendencies. The tensile stresses that cause fracture generally, therefore, are not caused by tensile loads (or traction) but rather by bending and torsion. These two phenomena are discussed in Chapter 1, Sections 8 and 10 and are taken up again in this chapter.

It is controversial as to whether plastic flow ever occurs in bone. "Greenstick" fracture is sometimes cited as an example of plastic flow in bone. However, greensticking could well represent a combination of small incomplete cracks or microfracture of one cortex of an immature poorly calcified bone which has a low modulus of elasticity. Certainly, in the laboratory, conditions can be created which can make bones plastically flow, but whether such conditions occur physiologically with any significant frequency is not known.

2. TENSILE STRESSES IN THE LONG BONES: BENDING AND TORSION

Significant stresses on bones are generated just by the activities of daily living. Consider stair climbing: body weight causes stresses on the bones of the legs as we propel ourselves upward against gravity. The force to move the body weight up the stairs is provided by muscle contraction. The bones are stressed as the muscles contract, bringing their origins and insertions closer together to move the joints. Thus the bony skeleton of the limbs is subjected to asymmetric com-

43

pression. Bending is the result. Any eccentric or off-center load creates bending and so the tibia, femur, and fibula are all subjected to bending stress when we go up stairs. The same is true when we walk. Additional asymmetric forces are caused by the relative position of the limbs visàvis the body weight (Fig. 2.1).

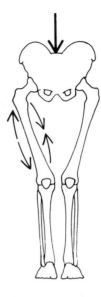

Figure 2.1. Asymmetric loading on the femur causes bending stresses.

Even without motion, double leg stance creates a bending stress in the lower extremity as the body weight is asymmetrically placed relative to the leg. The point at which body weight is centered (at which the body would balance on a pin) is called the *center of gravity*. In the human the center of gravity is just in front of the second sacral vertebra.

It has been calculated that the stresses during walking generated by the muscles on the hip, considered in and of themselves, are sufficient to bend the femoral neck permanently. Similar calculations can be made for the long bones of the upper extremity. Enormous forces can build up with isometric contractions, as in using one hand to oppose a forceful push by the other. Diseased bone frequently fractures, and normal bone subjected to impact loads can fracture, but the amazing thing is that normal bone doesn't continually fracture subjected to rather substantial bending stresses brought about by the activities of daily living. We now discuss why such disasters do not generally occur.

Fig. 2.2 illustrates the tensile and compressive stresses caused by long bone bending. As discussed in the preceding chapter, a bent structure has a neutral axis. The material on the concave side of the neutral axis is in compression and that on the convex side in tension. Thus, there is an important tension component in bending. In a solid such as bone, tension is a more potentially destructive stress than is compression. It is tensile stress that initiates fracture in bending (Fig. 2.3) and in most other common situations as well.

Many factors contribute to the resistance of bone to bending and in general keep the skeleton intact during normal physical activity. An uncontrolled or

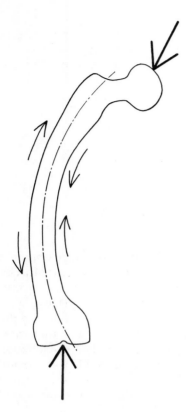

Figure 2.2. Bending stresses are tensile on the convex side and zero at the center line (neutral axis). (Strictly speaking, the neutral axis is a "center of gravity" and needn't be at the center line.)

substantial fall or high velocity impact is generally necessary to break a normal bone.

One of the primary mechanisms for stress relief operating in the appendicular skeleton is comprised of the articulations. Instead of our limbs bending in mid-shaft, most of the bending takes place at the joints, like articulations in the roadway of a bridge. Rather than the relatively rigid roadway bending, the articulations rotate (Fig. 2.4).

Some muscles also function to reduce bending stresses in bone. First they can act as "guy wires" to reduce bending. (Guy wires are familiar devices used to hold up high antennas and telephone poles.) In doing this the muscles increase the

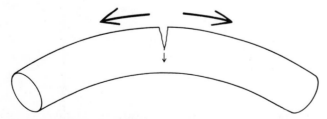

Figure 2.3. Fracture in bending always begins on the tensile side.

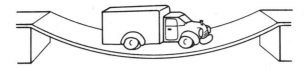

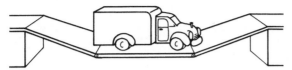

Figure 2.4. Articulations reduce bending in each section of the road.

compressive stress which for these purposes is not a disadvantage since bone has a greater resistance to fracture in compression than it does in tension. Muscles that straddle joints reduce bending stress by acting as guy wires and supporting part of the bones so that the entire bone is not subjected to bending (Fig. 2.5).

Biaxial muscles, which cross two joints, are even more effective in reducing the bending stress on bone. An added advantage of biaxial muscles is that most activities of daily living require combinations of joint actions, such as dorsiflexion of the wrist with flexion of the fingers or plantar flexion of the ankle with flexion of the knee. Such an arrangement of biaxial muscles makes maximal use of them and helps, in part, to explain the functional advantages in the rather complicated biaxial arrangement of so many muscles in the appendicular skeleton.

The structure of bone itself is designed to minimize bending stress. Bones are curved in order to be in line with the predominating resultant force which acts on them, increasing their compressive stress but decreasing their tendency to be bent (with its concomitant tension) (Fig. 2.6). Again there is a trade-off of tension for compression.

The hollow tubular structure of bone effectively reduces and resists bending, because the highest stress and, more importantly, the longest lever arm in longitudinal configurations subjected to bending is at the extreme outer fibers (refer

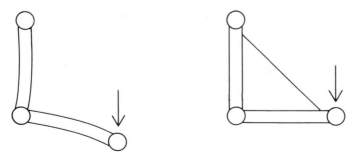

Figure 2.5. Muscle force introduces stresses opposite to the load, canceling much of the bending stresses and reducing the overall stress.

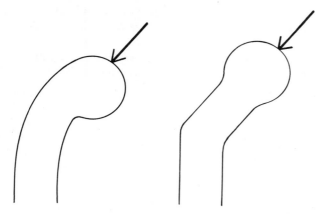

Figure 2.6. Each shape reduces bending at the end of the bone: the force is now lined up with the neutral axis and has no bending moment in the epiphyseal region.

to Chapter 1, Section 8). Stress becomes progressively less in the direction of the neutral fiber, which by definition is subjected to no bending stress. Thus material in direct proximity to the neutral fiber is of little use in strengthening the longitudinal structures against bending. Bones are hollow with little mass near their centers and most mass at the extreme outer fibers where the leverage and the stresses in bending are the greatest. A hollow shape provides bone with the maximum resistance to bending with the minimum of material.

Although bones are irregular in shape, the neutral axis can be located, with some effort. Once the neutral axis has been located the relative resistance to bending in a particular plane can be calculated. Thus each bone has a resistance to bending which increases with the mass out at the extreme fiber or, in other words, the mass multiplied by its lever arm to the neutral axis. This can be quantitated and is referred to as the *area moment of inertia*. Each bone, along its predominant bending axis, has an area moment of inertia which depends upon its geometry and distribution of mass relative to that geometry.*

The tubular cross-section of long bones facilitates circulation, repair, and nutrition, because two surfaces with osteogenic potency are available rather than one, and the hard tissue thickness which must be penetrated by osteoclasts, Haversian canals, and associated blood vessels is much reduced by the tubular shape.

All activities such as standing, walking, carrying, throwing, and pounding produce a predominant tensile stress on the convex side of the long bones as bending stresses are created within the bone. In gait, at foot flat, the maximum tensile stress on the tibia is posterior. The predominant tensile side of the femur is lateral, because it deviates back into the body from the intertrochanteric area, so that our knees almost touch (Fig. 2.1) All the large bones are acted on by many muscle groups as levers, and levers are always subjected to bending. Thus bend-

*In gross approximation, the material in a bone resists bending as the cube of its distance from the neutral axis. This value gives some idea of tremendous difference in strength achieved by even a small increment further out from the neutral axis.

ing is the predominant stress in the bones of the upper extremity as well. In the act of throwing, pounding, lifting, or carrying the predominant tensile side of the humerus and forearm bones is posterior (Fig. 2.7). As shown later in this chapter, knowledge of the predominant tensile and compressive side of long bone is important in considering the optimal placement of internal fixation devices and bone grafts.

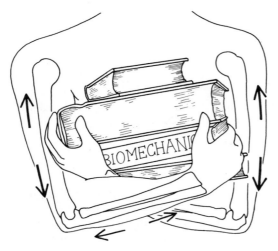

Figure 2.7. The posterior humeral, ulnar, and radial surfaces have the highest tensile stresses in most situations.

It has been shown by placing strain gauges on human and animal bones during gait and stance that the bones do bend and that the bending strain involved is physiologic. Remember that although bending is the predominant stress long bones are subjected to, they are also subjected to compression and to torsion. As in bending there is an important tensile component in torsion, as the next section shows. As in bending there is a neutral axis in torsion and the resistance to torsion depends upon the distance of the extreme fiber from its neutral axis. Again, this material has the greatest lever arm. As in bending the distribution of this material can be quantitated. This value for torsional resistance is known as the *polar moment of inertia* and for long bones approximates the fourth power of the distance of the material from the neutral axis. Thus the hollow structure of long bones is maximally effective to reduce torsion as well as bending.

3. MECHANICS OF FRACTURE: TENSILE STRESS AND STRESS CONCENTRATIONS

Fracture is very much a matter of the distribution of stress and mechanical energy. For instance, the work necessary to fracture the average human tibia is only about 1/10,000 of the kinetic energy of an 80 kg skier at 10 m/sec (24 mph).

Disaster occurs only when the kinetic energy is abruptly (and painfully) concentrated and converted to the work necessary to strain the tibia; even then, as we shall see, certain types of strain are far more harmful than others.

The stresses that occur in bending are discussed in Chapter 1. In bending, as Fig. 2.3 shows, the fracture should begin at the convex surface, at the extreme fiber with the highest tensile stress. If any grooves or scratches or other such features are on the extreme fiber, the crack begins at that point. In any case, the crack proceeds across the bar, perpendicular to the tensile stresses caused by the bending, as shown in Fig. 2.3. Transverse fractures of long bones are obviously due to bending. However, spiral fractures are due to torsion or twisting forces.

As shown in Fig. 2.8, twisting or applying torsion to a log of wood subjects it to shear strains (and stresses) in the horizontal plane. As twisting proceeds, note that the longitudinal fibers are stretched by the distortions due to the shearing. The fibers are also shearing in a nearly vertical direction, but neither the horizontal nor the vertical shearing is as critical as the stretching or tensile deformation. It is possible to show that the tensile stress is maximal at a 45° angle to the axis of torsion, and, as shown in Fig. 2.8, the fracture occurs at this angle. The fracture crack in many cases continues at this angle, and thus describes a 45° helix. The result is the so-called "spiral" fracture.

In most rigid materials, then, the fact that tensile stress causes fracture leads to transverse fracture when bending forces are applied and spiral fractures when torsional forces are applied. The exceptions to this rule are for very *anisotropic* materials, such as wood, in which the structure and the properties are highly directional. Bone, similar to wood in this respect, has planes of strength and planes of weakness: any long bone is much stronger in tension along its shaft than in tension in a transverse or tangential direction.

The cases of true bending or torsion are relatively simple. In any case, however complicated, there is always at any point a maximum shear stress on one plane and a maximum tensile stress on some other plane. In some cases in which

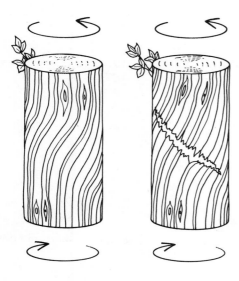

Figure 2.8. The highest tensile stress is on a plane 45° from the highest shear stress. In torsion the fracture crack tends to follow a spiral plane to maintain this angle.

there is little tensile stress but considerable shear stress fracture is inhibited and plastic flow occurs first. For instance, bending or torsion may be carried out in a fluid under large pressures; net tensile stresses may not even exist in such cases, and then even solids with a high resistance to plastic flow (such as extremely brittle materials) and solids which ordinarily shatter without deforming (such as glass) may deform under such circumstances.

On the other hand, in some circumstances tensile stresses are high and shear stresses low. Then, even materials that normally deform easily without breaking—*ductile* materials—may fracture catastrophically. Thus it is always important, in any mechanical situation involving failure, to assess the relative magnitudes of shear and tensile stresses.

Tensile stresses can be quite high at a *stress concentration*. Consider Fig. 2.9, in which the cross-section of a bar changes suddenly; the bar is loaded so as to be in tension. In mechanical equilibrium the total load is the same for any cross-section, so the stress must be higher in the narrow end of the bar, in inverse proportion to the ratio of the cross-sectional areas. To represent the stress, we use lines of force in Fig. 2.9: so many lines per cross-sectional area correspond to so many newtons per square meter, and the total number of lines is proportional to the total load on the bar. Thus, for mechanical equilibrium, each cross-section

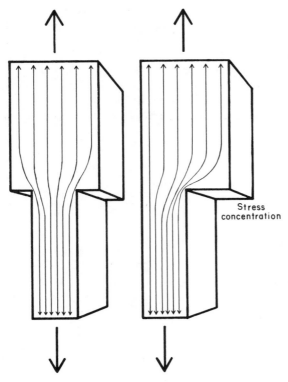

Stress
concentration

Figure 2.9. Stress is concentrated by sudden change in cross-section, at sharp interior corners.

must contain the same number of lines. A remarkable situation in the immediate vicinity of the change in section is a great concentration of stress, as shown by the concentration of the density of lines. Although the exact computation of the stress concentration requires use of the mathematical theory describing elasticity, stress concentrations can be measured by a variety of techniques and have been calculated for a number of common cases such as holes or notches in plates.

In Fig. 2.10 we show two ubiquitous geometric figures in which large stress concentrations occur. Holes, notches, grooves, threads, keyways, any change in section—all these (and many more!) serve to concentrate the stress. In a sharp, deep crack, tensile stresses may be concentrated by a factor of 10,000! As it turns out, solid materials of any kind contain a huge variety of microscopic defects, scratches, cracks, pores, etc. which can have sharp tips. *Brittle* materials (eg, glass) are readily cut by scribing a sharp scratch on the surface and then loading so that there is a tensile stress across the scratch. If such a scratch exists at the bottom of a thread or at a hole or cross-sectional change where the stress is concentrated, fracture may occur at low loads.

Because stress concentrations and some kinds of defects are unavoidable, in most cases solid stuctures would be much weaker than they are if the stress at the tip of a crack or scratch were the only factor that determined the likelihood of failure. Even if the local stress concentration were millions of newtons per

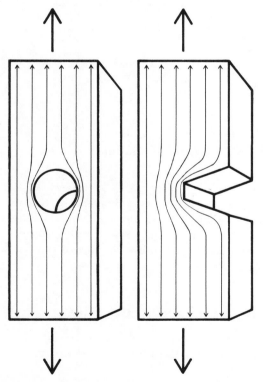

Figure 2.10. Stress is concentrated at the equator of the hole and at the bottom of the notch. A sharp notch would concentrate the stress further.

square inch, enough to rend apart the chemical bonds at the crack tip, the crack does not progress unless there is enough energy to push it along. The energy is necessary because the fracturing of material creates new surfaces, and the creation of new surface means the rupturing of chemical bonds which requires energy; per unit area, so many ergs (or calories or BTU's) of energy are needed, and this quantity is called the *surface energy* or "surface tension."

The applied forces supply the necessary energy for the creation of new surfaces. New surface is created by the growth of the crack. The occurrence of fracture then depends on a balance between the available mechanical energy and the energy needed to make the crack grow. The fracture stress for crack growth is also related to the initial depth of surface crack or scratch.* Deeper cracks weaken the material more drastically: The square of the stress required for fracture is inversely proportional to the crack depth. Thus, doubling the crack depth decreases fracture strength by nearly 30%. On the other hand, increased stiffness (Young's modulus) or surface energy increases the resistance to fracture.

In these discussions we have assumed that the applied tensile stress is perpendicular to the crack. As Fig. 2.11 shows, if the tensile stress is parallel to the crack, the crack does not spread. (In fact, the spreading of the crack has no effect on the parallel case: we should end up with two fragments with no change in stress.) If the crack is at some angle to the direction of the tensile stress, then we should consider the component of the stress which is perpendicular to the crack.

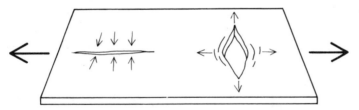

Figure 2.11. Crack perpendicular to the tensile stress opens and spreads, leading to fracture if the stress is sufficient.

As expected, larger cracks are "weaker." As any object contains an assortment of cracks or potential cracks (for example, lacunae, canaliculae, Haversian canals, and cement lines in bone), fracture is a matter of the "weakest link," that is, the largest crack giving way. Compressive stresses should not encourage the growth of cracks, but rather retard such processes.

4.   ENERGETICS OF FRACTURE, FRACTURE TOUGHNESS, AND IMPACT

The preceding discussion really describes the behavior of *brittle* materials. By "brittle" we mean a material that does not deform plastically or by viscous flow

---

*The general relation for fracture of a brittle material is

$$(\text{fracture stress})^2 = \frac{(4 \times \text{Young's modulus} \times \text{surface energy})}{(\text{depth of crack})}$$

prior to fracture; typically, very hard materials are intrinsically brittle, as they do not deform until high stresses (well above the fracture stress) are reached.

Suppose the stress versus strain behavior of two materials are plotted, as in Fig. 2.12. The work (per unit volume) to fracture each material is simply the total area under its tensile curve. Thus the soft, annealed copper requires much more work to fracture it than the extremely hard carbide tool material. The work required to fracture a material is referred to as fracture *toughness*.

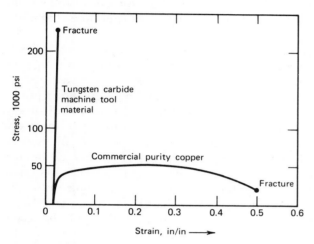

Figure 2.12. Stress versus strain for a soft, ductile material (copper) and a hard, brittle material (tungsten carbide).

One reason why softer materials may be tougher may be seen by considering what happens at the tip of a crack under stress in such a material (eg, stainless steel): the large stresses at the crack tip cause local viscous or plastic flow. As a result, more work must be absorbed by the crack: the material near the crack is severely deformed. This work must be added to the surface energy. Thus ductility, however small, increases the fracture stress. Consequently, impact causes failure much more readily. The effect is further amplified because a fracture crack accelerates if the energy to do so is available; however, once acceleration occurs, less energy is needed to propagate the crack and further acceleration is inevitable. On the other hand, if for some reason the crack slows down, more energy is needed to continue, and the crack decelerates until it stops.

5.   FATIGUE FRACTURE; "MARCH" FRACTURES; RESISTANCE OF CORTICAL BONE TO FRACTURES

Even at low stress levels, far below the stresses necessary to cause catastrophic failure or observable viscous or plastic flow, the seeds of failure may be sown. The most common type of loading is cyclic or intermittent; locomotion puts repetitive or cyclic stresses on the lower extremities. Even if the stress is well below the fracture stress so that a pre-existing crack does not immediately grow, there may be enough to advance it a few microns. Each time the stress is reapplied, the crack advances another few microns. Eventually the crack is large enough to increase catastrophically. Such a phenomenon is called "*fatigue* failure." We have illustrated this process in Fig. 2.13, with a scanning electron micrograph which shows the markings left by the crack; each "fatigue striation" in the micrograph marks the place where the crack stopped and then resumed its growth.

The larger the intermittent or cyclic stress, the farther the crack advances with each application, as shown in Fig. 2.14. Thus the larger the cyclic stresses, the faster the rate of growth, and the final failure occurs in a shorter time, that is, the "fatigue life" is shorter.

In Fig. 2.15 we present typical fatigue data, where the number of cycles to cause failure is plotted as a function of the maximum stress applied during each cycle; variation of stress with time is also illustrated.

For many materials there is a stress level below which the fatigue life is practically infinite; this stress level is called the *fatigue limit* and is indicated in Fig. 2.15B for steel. Obviously the fatigue limit is a good number to stay below in any mechanical design. However, if stress concentrations are present, this may be impossible. This, then, is by far the most common history of mechanical failure: first, a stress concentration occurs, through defective design, defective materials, accidents, or careless operation or handling; from the stress concentration, a fatigue crack slowly grows; when the fatigue crack has grown large enough, the final catastrophic failure occurs. It is often possible to determine with the naked eye this course of events by examining the fracture surfaces, as in Fig. 2.16, because the textures left by fatigue and catastrophic propagation are different.

It is possible that fatigue failure of bone is important in some cases as, for

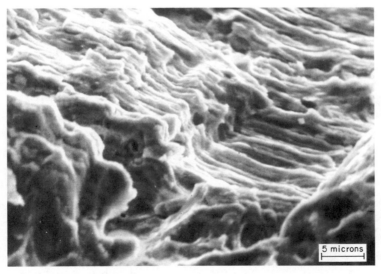

Figure 2.13. Fatigue striations on the fracture surface of a fractured Schneider pin. The striations are ¼ to ½ micron wide (1 micron = 10^{-4} cm).

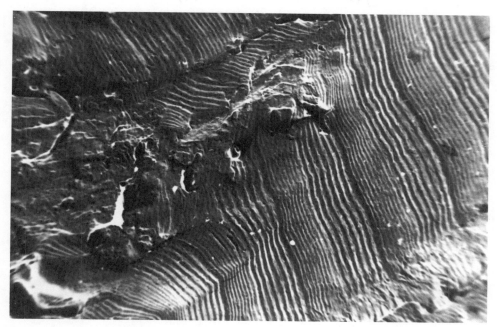

Figure 2.14. Striations (less than a micron wide) produced in a fatigue testing machine programmed to produce seven cycles at high stress and then seven cycles at low stress, repeatedly. The striations are therefore in groups of seven, wide and narrow, since higher stress produces larger striations. (Courtesy RMN Pelloux.)

example, "march fractures." Bone with a higher density of Haversian systems has a greater fatigue resistance. This is probably so because the cement lines and Haversian canals serve to divert and arrest the growth of the crack. The subdivision of bone by cement lines tends to guide the crack longitudinally; however, if the osteons tend to bend individually, there is less rigidity in bending.

The Haversian canals also help to prevent fracture, as shown in Figs. 2.17 and

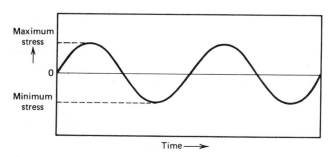

Figure 2.15A. Time-varying loading cycle that is often used to determine the fatigue test, maximum tensile stress reached during one portion of the cycle is equal to the maximum compressive stress reached during the other portion of the cycle when the load is reversed.

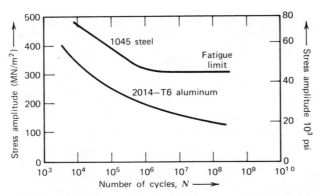

Figure 2.15B. Experimentally determined stress versus number of cycles curves for a plain-carbon steel (0.47% carbon) and an age-hardened aluminum alloy. These curves are for fully reversed stresses (see Fig. 2.15A). The steel shows a fatigue limit, that is, a stress below which it will not fail regardless of the number of cycles. The aluminum alloy shows no fatigue limit, but the slope of stress vs log N becomes less negative as the stress decreases. (Adapted from Hayden HW, Moffatt WG, Wulff J: *The Structure and Properties of Materials*, vol 3: *Mechanical Behavior.* New York, John Wiley & Sons, 1965.)

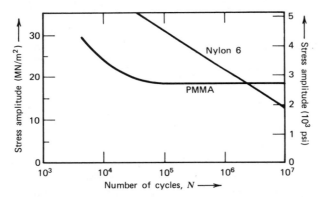

Figure 2.15C. Stress versus number of cycles curves for the polymers nylon and PMMA (Lucite). Lucite shows a fatigue limit, but nylon does not. (After Riddell MN, Koo GP, O'Toole JL: *Polymer Eng Sci* 6:363, 1966.)

2.18. The canal has a much larger radius of curvature, that is, it is not as "sharp" as the crack edge, so that much higher stresses are required to resume propagation of the crack. (In the early days of aviation, it is said that the precaution against fatigue failure of the wing was to drill holes in the probable path of the crack!) On the other hand, for march fractures, another kind of fatigue is also probably important, and that is fatigue of muscles that act to reduce the tensile stresses due to bending of the long bones, as discussed earlier.

The ultrastructure of bone is also remarkable in mechanical properties. On the finest scale of observation (electron microscope), bone consists of a highly ordered protein (collagen) matrix reinforced with mineral (hydroxyapatite, $Ca_{10}[PO_4]_6[OH]_2$) crystals. Collagen is known to be a relatively soft, pliable

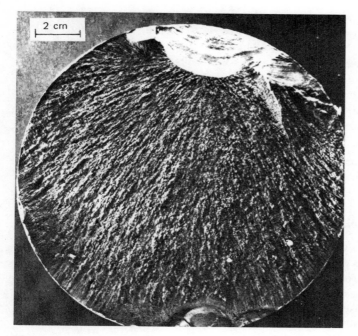

Figure 2.16. Macrostructure of a fatigue failure surface of a steel piston rod. Fracture originated at the top edge. The smooth area, with the "clamshell" markings, corresponds to slow fatigue crack growth, and the dull fibrous section is the region of fast fracture. (From *Metals Handbook,* vol 9, ed 8. American Society for Metals, 1974.)

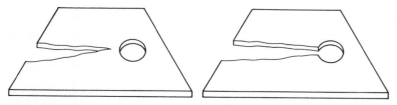

Figure 2.17. Advancing crack blunted and stopped by a hole.

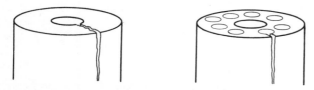

Figure 2.18. Haversian systems may resist fracture in the same way as shown in Fig. 2.17.

material; the mechanical properties of soft connective tissue typify collagen. Bone mineral, as observed in vitro, is brittle and friable, resembling chalk in mechanical properties. Neither the collagen nor the mineral would serve satisfactorily as a skeletal structural material by itself: collagen is not stiff enough and the mineral is too brittle. However, the composite material, with fine crystals of mineral (about 0.05 micron long and 0.005 micron wide) embedded in the protein matrix has excellent mechanical properties, similar to those of teak wood. (In fact, the properties of bone are superior in that there is less directionality or "grain".)

6.   CORROSION OF METALLIC IMPLANTS

Many commercial alloys with extremely high strength would be useful in fixation devices and prostheses but are unacceptable because of inadequate *corrosion* resistance. Corrosion products can, in the extreme, cause bone necrosis and "rust granulomas" in the adjacent soft tissues; in less severe cases, pain and inflammation may occur under aseptic conditions. Many designs and materials now in use are in fact marginal with regard to corrosion resistance, and care should be exercised in their use, as discussed below.

As Fig. 2.19 shows, the driving force for corrosion is also the basis of the

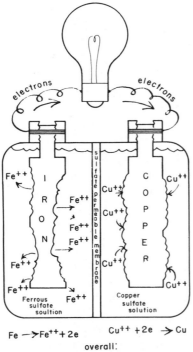

$$Fe \rightarrow Fe^{++} + 2e \qquad Cu^{++} + 2e \rightarrow Cu$$

overall:

$$Fe + Cu^{++} \rightarrow Fe^{++} + Cu$$

Figure 2.19. Battery based on the reaction Fe + $Cu^{++} \rightarrow Fe^{++}$ + Cu. The iron corrodes and is ultimately dissolved.

electrical storage battery: the energy released by a chemical reaction may be used to drive electrons through a circuit or device and do useful work, but only at the cost of exhausting the battery by partially or completely consuming one of the reactants. The consumption, when it occurs unintentionally, is commonly referred to as corrosion. If an iron nail is dipped into copper sulfate solution a reddish deposit appears on the nail. The deposit is copper, which is displaced from the solution by the reaction:

$$Fe + Cu^{++} \rightarrow Fe^{++} + Cu$$

In general, a more active metal always displaces a less active (or more "noble") metal from solution. We could, if we wanted to, arrange to have the electrons transferred from the iron to the cupric ion through a wire rather than directly; the resulting device would be a battery (with a maximum voltage of about 3/4 volt).

Thus, corrosion occurs due to differences in chemical reactivity, which gives rise to electrical currents generated by destruction of the more reactive material. The example used in Fig. 2.19 is based on reactivity differences due to dissimilar metals. However, even the same metal has different reactivity in a different environment. A common environmental difference that can cause corrosion is a different oxygen concentration and this can occur in a body fluid or in water. In a situation such as that shown in Fig. 2.20, with identical iron electrodes but a higher concentration of dissolved oxygen on one side, the reduction reaction has

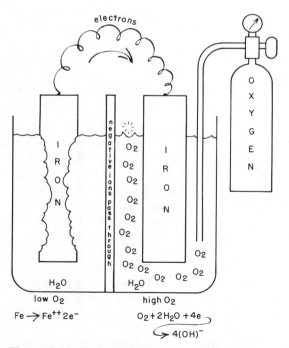

Figure 2.20. Battery based on a difference in oxygen concentration. The iron electrode in the *low* oxygen side corrodes.

greater "reactivity" on the oxygen-rich side. Therefore, the following reaction occurs on the side with higher oxygen:

$$O_2 + 2H_2O + 4e^- \rightarrow 4(OH)^-$$

The reaction on the "oxygen-poor" side is:

$$Fe \rightarrow Fe^{++} + 2e^-$$

As before, the electrons generated by the oxidation reaction (on the left side in Fig. 2.20) are fed through the electrical connection to the reduction reaction, on the right side of the cell in Fig. 2.20.

Thus, differences in oxygen concentration can lead to corrosion, and the damage occurs where the least oxygen is. The most extensive corrosion occurs underneath the heads of screws and other fasteners rather than on top: the screw head itself has free access to the oxygen around it, but just beneath the screw head, it is more difficult for oxygen to penetrate. Consider Fig. 2.21, which shows the most likely areas of corrosive attack on a bone plate: all areas are exposed to seepage of body fluids, but access to dissolved oxygen is slight. This is called crevice corrosion, and is by far the most common type in surigcal implants.

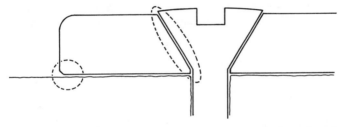

Figure 2.21. Probable sites for "crevice" corrosion based on the oxygen concentration cell shown in Fig. 2.20.

Fig. 2.22 is a clinical example: This plate had to be removed because corrosion under the screw heads and the edges of the plate were causing considerable pain.

There is another dimension to this problem: stainless steels and the other alloys used in orthopedic implants all are so effective against corrosion because continuous, tightly bound oxide films are on their surfaces; the alloys themselves, if perfectly clean, are quite reactive. This reactivity binds the protective film tightly. Nitric acid makes the films even better. However, chloride ions puncture the film. In the body, of course, Cl^- is readily available, and even with the low H^+ levels present many alloys that are considered very resistant to corrosion become rapidly and extensively pitted due to failure of the protective films.

Finally, there is some evidence that the metal ions liberated at the *anode* portion of the crevice hydrolyze the water in the vicinity. In physiologic media, then, each corroding crevice is a veritable HCl generator!

To make it worse, stress concentrations may occur at crevices, and stress always makes metals more reactive. A stress concentration alone can create an

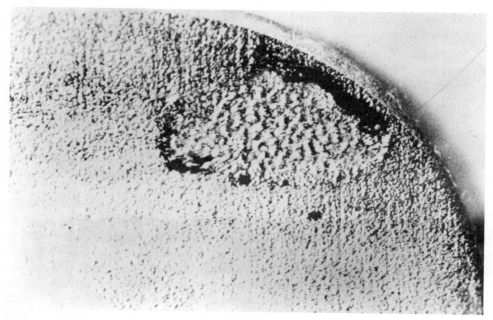

Figure 2.22. Corrosion at the edge of a bone plate, as shown schematically in Fig. 2.21. (Courtesy of J Cohen.)

anode and cause corrosion; together with the oxygen concentration difference between the inside and outside of the crevice, the effect is reinforced.

Finally, consider corrosion pits on a previously smooth surface as stress concentrators that can start fatigue cracks; also that the stress concentration at the crack tip accelerates corrosion, as does the "crevice" or oxygen concentration effect. Obviously, corrosion can drastically accelerate fatigue failure. (In practice, fatigue life in a corrosive environment may fall to 1/1000 or less of its former value.) Also, the paramount importance of avoiding stress concentrations and optimizing corrosion resistance is apparent. To achieve the latter:

- use resistant alloys.
- avoid dissimilar metals.
- avoid ion concentration difference.
- avoid oxygen concentration differences including crevices.
- avoid stress concentrations.

7. IMPLANT MATERIALS FOR INTERNAL FIXATION DEVICES

In general, the following are straightforward rules for selecting and making an orthopedic implant:

- The material and design should have adequate mechanical strength and fatigue resistance. Since bone has tensile strength of (roughly) 70 million newtons/m² (10,000 psi) and a compressive strength of about twice that number, and the size of the implant is restricted, the material should tolerate stresses of 700 million newtons/m² (100,000 psi).

● Corrosion resistance should be extremely good.

● There should be no toxic, carcinogenic, or allergenic reaction.

In fact, as shown in the next section, the mechanical functions of most implants involve tensile stresses in particular, and therefore the tensile properties are of greatest interest. A familiar engineering test of tensile properties is the *tensile* test described in Fig. 2.23: a specimen is strained at a constant rate, and the stress recorded as a function of strain. (Alternatively, the load could be slowly increased and the strain measured as a function of stress).

Several features of importance in the tensile test data are shown in Fig. 2.24. First, the stress at which permanent plastic deformation occurs is called the *yield stress* or *yield strength*—generally taken as the stress at which the specimen is permanently stretched 0.2%. Since the specimen is also stretching elastically, it is necessary to use the elastic (Young's) modulus to subtract the elastic strain from the total strain as the test continues, in order to identify the yield point. After yielding, the material may, if it is ductile, continue to deform, usually with increasing stress, until a maximum stress, the *ultimate tensile stress,* is reached.

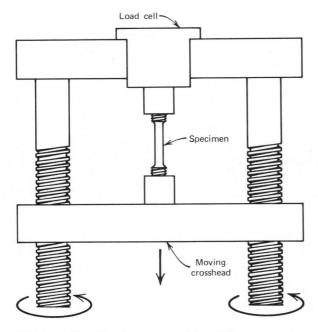

Figure 2.23. Tensile test machine. The two screws drive the horizontal bars apart, stretching the specimen. The load cell measures stress. The strain can be measured with a mechanical gauge. (From Hayden HW, Moffatt WG, Wulff J: *The Structure and Properties of Materials,* vol 3: *Mechanical Behavior.* New York, John Wiley & Sons, 1965.)

This is the second feature of general interest. Finally, when strained sufficiently, the material fractures. The strain or *elongation at fracture* is the third feature of general interest as it indicates the ductility of the material.

As the tensile curves in Figs. 2.12 and 2.24 show, some materials have very large elastic strains; some are so brittle they fracture before the yield point occurs, and others deform so easily that there really is no ultimate tensile stress. However, the metallic alloys used for implants generally exhibit all three features, and their relative values are used to compare the materials. Ideally, all three data, the yield stress, ultimate tensile stress, and elongation at fracture should be as large as possible. In practice, some trade-offs between strength and ductility have to be made. The requirement for high ultimate tensile strength (about 700 million newtons/m²) has in the past restricted the choice of structural materials for fixation and prosthetic devices to metallic alloys. Future possibilities such as strong ceramics and polymeric fiber composites are being investigated. At present five metallic alloys are in general use:

Stainless Steel

Stainless steels have been used for implants for about 40 years. The best stainless alloy for surgical use is type 316L, which has 17 to 20% chromium, 10 to 14 % nickel, 2 to 4% molybdenum, very low (less than 0.08%) carbon, and the rest iron. These alloys can be *forged,** and they harden (ie, the yield strength increases) as the amount of cold forging or plastic deformation increases, but at the same expense of some ductility. They can be made softer (weaker) and more ductile by annealing (heating in a suitable furnace). Thus, in severely forged 316L stainless steel the yield stress may be as high as 875 million newtons/m² (125,000 psi) with an elongation of 15% (or less) at fracture, whereas a thoroughly annealed piece of the same material may have a yield stress of 210 million newtons/m² (30,000 psi or less!) but an elongation of 50% or more.

For load bearing implants, forged material is generally required. Cast stainless steel is not as strong as forged stainless; yield stresses of 210 million newtons/m² or less are common for the cast material. In addition, the castings are chemically inhomogeneous and therefore have inferior corrosion resistance as well. Thus cast stainless steel is poorly suited to implant applications. Forged stainless steel has superior mechanical properties and is relatively low in cost. However, even the best 316L has only marginal in vivo corrosion resistance; it has been shown that in typical clinical applications of multicomponent implants (eg, plate with screws) some corrosion is inevitable in this material. Further, the corrosion resistance decreases as the strength increases, so that there is a compromise between mechanical properties and corrosion resistance.

Stainless steel is the material of choice for fixation devices which can be removed in a year or two.

Forging is essentially, in this particular context, the art of the blacksmith; the metal is heated and hammered or squeezed into shape. This may or may not be done with aid of a die which is a mold to guide the flow of the metal. Alternatively, metal may be shaped by casting (ie, melting and pouring into a mold) and subsequent solidification.

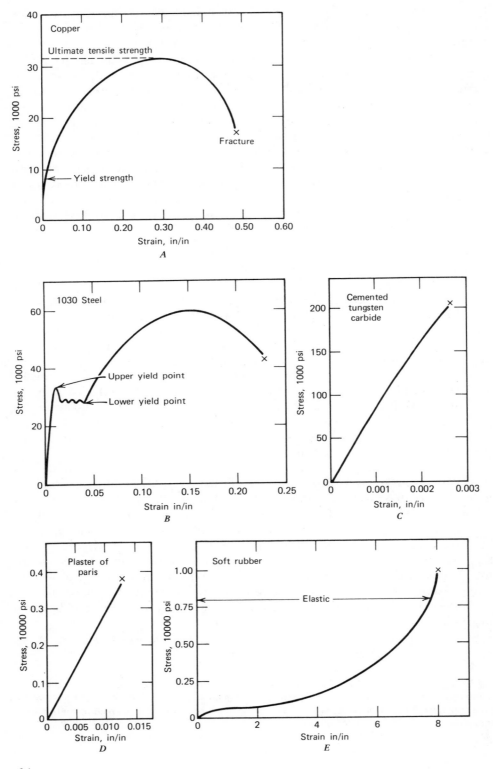

64

Cast Cobalt-Chromium-Molybdenum Alloy

This alloy was discovered 70 years ago and used for tools and similar applications. It was soon used for dental restorations and, about 40 years ago, for orthopedic implants, mainly fixation devices. The alloy's composition is 63 to 70% cobalt, 25 to 30% chromium, and 5 to 7% molybdenum, with minor amounts of impurities such as manganese, nickel, iron, and carbon. It is sold under various trade names.

It is much more resistant to in vivo corrosion than 316L stainless steel (or any other stainless steel). The chief disadvantage of the Co-Cr-Mo alloy is that its mechanical properties are inferior to those of stainless steel (see Table 2.1). The alloy is *cast* by a relatively expensive process and generates a variety of microscopic defects which limit its strength, ductility, and fatigue life. It is the material of choice for permanent implants because of its superior in vivo corrosion resistance and also because such implants can usually be more massive than fixation devices. The possibility of improving the mechanical properties of this alloy is the subject of considerable attention.

Wrought Cobalt-Chromium-Tungsten-Nickel Alloy

Discovered at about the same time as the cast Co-Cr-Mo alloy, the wrought alloy is 52 to 58% cobalt, 19 to 21% chromium, 14 to 16% tungsten, 9 to 11% nickel, and miscellaneous minor impurities. This alloy is much easier to forge than cast Co-Cr-Mo alloy. Its mechanical properties are approximately the same as 316L stainless steel and its corrosion resistance is intermediate, better than 316L stainless but inferior to the cast Co-Cr-Mo alloy discussed above. It is important not to confuse the wrought Co-Cr-W-Ni alloy with the cast Co-Cr-Mo alloy, as it is not good practice to combine them in multicomponent prostheses. For instance, nail-plate assemblies with plates of the wrought alloy and nails or screws of the cast alloy have been shown to corrode in vivo and cause clinical problems. Unfortunately this alloy has been sold under the same trade name(s) as the cast Co-Cr-Mo alloy.

Titanium

Commercially pure titanium is highly resistant to corrosion but has low yield and ultimate tensile stresses, and therefore is not considered to be generally suitable for fracture fixation devices.

Titanium "Six-Four" Alloy

This alloy has 5.5 to 6.5% aluminum and 3.5 to 4.5% vanadium in a titanium base, with few impurities permitted. The usual grade offered for implant fabri-

---

Figure 2.24. *A,* tensile test data for copper as usually plotted. Engineering stress-strain curves for several engineering materials: *B,* 1030 steel. *C,* cemented tungsten carbide. *D,* plaster of Paris. *E,* soft rubber. (From Hayden HW, Moffatt WG, Wulff J: *The Structure and Properties of Materials,* vol 3: *Mechanical Behavior.* New York, John Wiley & Sons, 1965.)

Table 2.1. Mechanical Properties of Implant Alloys

	316L Stainless Steel	Cast Co-Cr-Mo Alloy	Wrought Co-Cr-T-Ni Alloy	Titanium	Titanium "Six-Four" Alloy
Yield stress (N/m²)	$250\text{-}900 \times 10^6$	500×10^6	550×10^6	300×10^6	815×10^6
(psi)	35-125,000	70,000	78,000	40,000	145,000
Ultimate tensile stress (N/m²)	$560\text{-}1 \times 10^9$	700×10^6	1.1×10^9	350×10^6	1.2×10^9
(psi)	80-145,000	100,000	155,000	50,000	165,000
Elongation at fracture (%)	45-15	8.0	35	22	15

cation is the "ELI" grade, with specially low levels of carbon, oxygen, nitrogen, and hydrogen; not uncommonly the sum of these impurities is below 0.1% in such a grade. Such purity enhances ductility and resistance to fracture even in the presence of stress concentrations. This alloy, when forged and properly heat treated, has mechanical properties that are superior to all of the above-mentioned materials, and extreme resistance to crevice corrosion as well. (The cast version of this alloy is markedly inferior to the wrought version in mechanical properties, much as in the case of stainless steel.) Corrosion products of titanium appear to be less inflammatory than other metals. Since titanium alloys are recent arrivals compared to the other implant materials, some questions remain; however, the general clinical experience for the two decades these alloys have been implanted has been very good.

Table 2.1 compares the mechanical properties of the alloys discussed in this section. For the reasons discussed above, the most popular alternatives are cast Co-Cr-Mo and 316L stainless steel. The latter offers superior mechanical properties, low cost, and reliability (freedom from casting defects) but at the cost of corrosion resistance. A recent study of multicomponent stainless steel implants removed for various clinical reasons showed that more than 90% had corroded. Thus stainless steel should be used in fracture fixation devices that cannot be too massive and rigid, and therefore bear higher stresses and that can be removed after the fracture heals. For prosthetic implants or any device that must remain in place indefinitely, the cast Co-Cr-Mo alloy is the material of choice.

As Table 2.2 shows, high-strength engineering materials are much stiffer than bone. Thus, a fixation device made massive in order to avoid fatigue failure is also very stiff, and bears much more of the normal loads which would otherwise be taken up by the bone. Normal healing and remodeling of the bone would therefore be impeded. Thus proper fixation devices are limited in strength and should be regarded as essentially alignment aids and not be expected to bear full ambulatory loads for extended time periods. If nonunion occurs, fatigue failure of the device is inevitable. A clinical advantage of high-strength materials for fracture fixation is that the fatigue life is longer (at equivalent loads) and slowly healing fractures may be treated without fear of interruption by implant failure.

It is appropriate—especially in patients with normal bone—to remove the fracture fixation device as soon as healing is adequate, to allow the stresses generated by the activities of daily living to pass through the bone and stimulate remodeling. As long as the implant is present, much of the load is borne by the stiffer metal and the bone under the metal becomes osteopenic. Refracture is

Table 2.2. Young's Modulus of Bone and Typical Engineering Materials

	N/m^2	psi
Tungsten	395.5×10^9	56.5×10^6
Stainless steels	$196\text{-}210 \times 10^9$	$28\text{-}30 \times 10^6$
Titanium alloys	$105\text{-}119 \times 10^9$	$15\text{-}17 \times 10^6$
Bone: cortical	$7\text{-}21 \times 10^9$	$1\text{-}3 \times 10^6$
cancellous	$0.7\text{-}4.9 \times 10^9$	$0.1\text{-}0.7 \times 10^6$
Polymethyl methacrylate	$2.5\text{-}3.5 \times 10^9$	$0.35\text{-}0.5 \times 10^6$
Polyethylene	$0.14\text{-}0.42 \times 10^6$	$0.02\text{-}0.06 \times 10^6$

therefore most likely in the bone immediately adjacent to the end of a plate, as a result of stress concentration, and the osteopenic bone under the plate, as shown in Fig. 2.25.

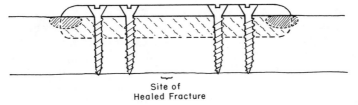

Site of
Healed Fracture

Figure 2.25. The plate lowers the stress in the adjacent bone (lightly shaded areas) leading to osteopenia. Furthermore, due to the discontinuity in stiffness there is a stress concentration at each end of the osteopenic region.

8.   MECHANICAL CONSIDERATIONS IN TREATMENT OF FRACTURES

Before considering internal fixation devices on fractured bones, let us consider mechanical factors involved in the functional treatment of fractures. Joint motion maintained through the period of fracture healing obviates the long term physical therapy frequently necessary to regain motion in a joint whose capsule has been immobilized for long periods of time and is scarred down. Also, intermittent loading speeds fracture healing. Whether this occurs by generating the electrical potentials which have been seen in bone subjected to intermittent loading or bending or is merely an incidental reflection of mechanical stress is not certain. Generation of electrical activity is a property common to almost all organic material and is the result of the fact that organic molecules may be asymmetric or may be arranged so as to have an asymmetric charge distribution.

Consider the two arrangements in Fig. 2.26: the positive and negative charges are symbolized by full and open circles, respectively. In B, the arrangement has no symmetry across the horizontal plane, and a voltage results as the material is compressed. A is symmetric across the plane of compression, and no voltage appears. Quartz crystals are essentially equivalent to the arrangement in B and are *piezoelectric*; rock salt, which is equivalent to the arrangement in A, is not. Whether this is meaningful physiologically or is just a coincidental physical happening is not clear, but there is no question that the application of intermittent load—whether it be electrical or physical—does speed fracture healing.

The relationship between metabolic activity and mechanical stress has been known for years. The older German literatures suggest that mesodermal (connective tissue) primitive cells subjected to pure tension and pure compression tend to form bone, as shown schematically in Fig. 2.27 .Similar cells subjected to shear form fibrous tissue and such cells under equal pressure (hydrostatic pressure) from all directions form cartilage. (The implications of this in the formation of reparative articular surfaces are discussed in Chapter 4.)

Thus, stress primarily in pure tension or pure compression and intermittent in nature aids in fracture healing. More recent observations indicate that certain amounts of motion are compatible with healing fractures and that actually some

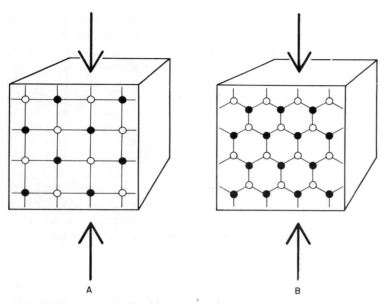

Figure 2.26. *A,* Schematic "rock salt" crystal: full circles represent Na+; open circles are Cl−. Across any horizontal plane there is symmetry; a sodium ion on one side is in a position identical to a sodium ion on the other. Thus, when the stress shifts the ions, all charge movements cancel and no voltage is induced. *B,* Crystal with no symmetry across the horizontal plane; a voltage is produced, that is, it is piezoelectric.

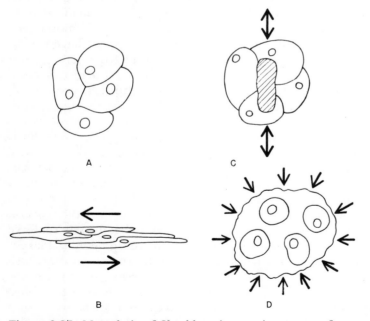

Figure 2.27. Metaplasia of fibroblasts into various types of connective tissue under the influence of mechanical stress has been reported. Primitive cells *(A)* under shear create fibrous tissue *(B)*: under pure tension or compression bone is formed *(C),* and hydrostatic pressure results in a cartilagenous matrix *(D).*

shear is permissible if it is small; apparently, limited shear aggravates the formation of fracture callus and more callus is laid down around fractures that have slight motion than those that are rigidly immobilized. Certainly significant shear or bending at fracture sites is clinically known to lead to nonunion and—if the motion is great enough—to formation of a pseudoarthrosis.

The most effective way to transmit a stress, which is limited in shear and bending (and, of course, torsion), but is mainly of tensile or compressive nature, is with a cast brace or weight-bearing cast. Tibial fractures submitted to weight-bearing in a cast brace heal two to three times faster than similar fractures treated in non-weight-bearing plasters or with the patient on crutches. Such cast-brace treatment is associated with proliferative callus which acts as a scaffold, immobilizing the fracture fragments. This method of fracture treatment is in marked contradistinction to rigid internal fixation where external callus formation is minimal and sometimes even nonexistent. Here again the basic principle is to eliminate bending and torsional stresses on the fracture site as much as possible.

9. INTERNAL FIXATION DEVICES: WIRE AND TENSION BANDS

As discussed above, the role of mechanical stress in the healing of fractures is incompletely known and in some respects controversial. However, satisfactory results are known to occur when the fracture fragments are in reasonable apposition and relative motion of the fragments is limited.

In general, muscular activity tends to bring fracture fragments together. In certain places on bone, individual muscles can act to separate fragments, such as the iliopsoas tendon, pulling the entire lower extremity below the femoral neck fracture into external rotation. But, in general, tensile forces, as we have seen in our discussion of fracture mechanisms, result physiologically from bending and torsional stress, also due to muscle forces. The purpose of fracture fixation devices is therefore alignment and resistance to tensile stress. Therefore, all fracture fixation devices can be considered as bands that resist tension and are most effective if placed on the tensile side of the fracture.

The simplest demonstration of this general principle in internal fixation is wire fixation. Consider the wiring of a patella fracture (Fig. 2.28). The wire serves to tie together opposing points on the anterior cortex about the point of contact, and a torque equilibrium is maintained for the distal fragment, as shown in Fig. 2.28 for a small angle of flexion. The moment of the tendon force is balanced by the reaction force from the other fragment: note that the reaction force is compressive. In other words, the wire is attached so that the tendon force rotates the distal fragment into contact with the proximal fragment, and larger tendon forces cause larger compressive forces across the fracture surface. All this occurs provided that contact at the fulcrum (the anterior cortex) is maintained by tension in the wire. The reaction force and the tendon force both have appreciable components in the same direction, which can only be balanced by a tensile force in the wire; thus the phrase *tension band*. An analogous situation with two pieces of hardware connected by a hinge is also shown in Fig. 2.28.

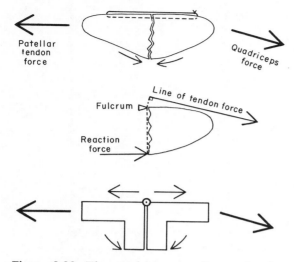

Figure 2.28. The quadriceps–patellar tendon forces produce compression in the fragments when the anterior cortex is wired.

Another example is wire fixation of the olecranon process of the elbow, as shown in Fig. 2.29. The wire anchors the two fragments together as close to the outer surface as possible, so that the triceps force rotates the two fragments together, and keeps them together with a compressive reaction force, which is required in order to maintain torque equilibrium about the "hinge," that is, the point of contact maintained by the wire. By considering full force equilibrium in the horizontal direction, we can see that the compressive reaction force must be balanced by an equal and opposite force in the wire, a tensile force as shown in Fig. 2.30.

Properly done, the wire method is much more effective than using a screw. As shown in Fig. 2.31, with screw fixation the "hinge" or center of rotation is no longer at the central portion of the fracture. Thus, the outer portion of the fracture, as shown by the "hardware" analogue, is free to open up when the triceps force is applied; this tendency is counteracted only partially by the rigidity of the screw. In addition, the screw is subjected to bending stresses. Screws are not designed (nor intended) to withstand significant bending stresses, and the latter should be avoided or minimized.

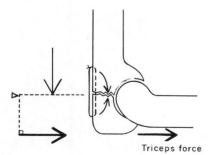

Triceps force

Figure 2.29. Correct wiring of the olecranon converts muscle forces into compression.

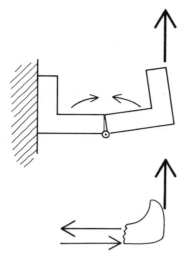

Figure 2.30. A mechanical analogy to the forces on the olecranon in Fig. 2.29.

10. INTERNAL FIXATION DEVICES: PLATES

A multiple-screw plate, mounted on the extreme fiber in tension of a long bone, is similar in some respects to the wire fixation cases discussed above. As Fig. 2.32 shows, if the plate is properly located, bending moments lead to compressive forces across the fracture. In this case, although the plate participates in bending because it is at the extreme fiber, the stress in the plate is essentially tensile in nature (as in the case of wire fixation) for the ideal case of perfect apposition. The screws serve to constrain the bone-plate composite system so that they do in fact act together in bending, with the plate in tension.

There are a number of complications and potential sources of difficulty in this arrangement. For instance, if the plate is not tightly set against the bone by the screws, but is offset, the screws may have bending stresses on them (Fig. 2.33). At least two screws are necessary on each side of the fracture to prevent rotation due to moments that may occur at right angles to the principal bending moment.

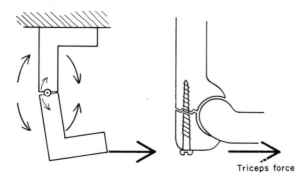

Triceps force

Figure 2.31. Screw fixation of the olecranon moves the pivot to the interior, so that only one side of the fracture is compressed by the muscle force.

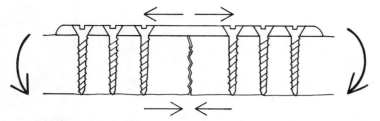

Figure 2.32. When the plate is located at the tensile surface, the fracture is compressed by the muscle forces across most or all of the fracture surface.

Since apposition is rarely (if ever) perfect, the plate is usually subjected, for some period of time, to a certain amount of bending with little or no assistance from the bone. Thus, if the plate is too thin, it fails in fatigue due to repeated bending. If a screw is omitted from a hole near the fracture, the plate may bend excessively at the empty screw hole, as it is not constrained to the bone there and the screw hole is a weak point; due to the stress concentration the result may well be fatigue failure at the screw hole.

One way to increase the supporting function of the bone and decrease the bending of the plate is to use a compression plate, a plate devised so as to put the fracture in compression even in the absence of forces or movements from the rest of the musculoskeletal system. Various mechanical devices and modifications are available to achieve this effect: specially shaped screw holes that force the screw (and therefore the bone) to move along the plate, toward the fracture side, as the screw is tightened; or devices that force the bone together in compression before the screw holes are drilled and the plate installed.

Each method has unique advantages and disadvantages, but all methods put the bone in compression and the plate in tension. Since the fracture surface is irregular, the compressive load is borne by a relatively small portion of the fracture surface, that is, by asperities in contact. After about 72 hours these asperities are resorbed and the compressive stress in the bone (and tensile stress in the plate) due to the compression device, has generally vanished. However, the apposition of the fracture is greatly improved in most cases, so that the ideal case shown in Fig. 2.32 is approached. With poor apposition the plate alone bears the bending moment, as in Fig. 2.33. Obviously, such a situation is not desirable. From the discussion in Chapter 1 on bending it is apparent that the plate alone in this situation has little rigidity compared to the plate-bone compo-

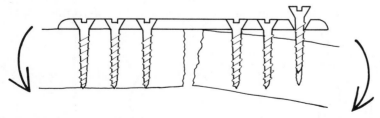

Figure 2.33. If the plate is not tightly fastened to the bone, bending stresses occur on the screws.

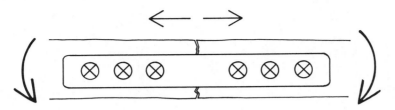

Figure 2.34. Arrangement 10 to 100 times as rigid as that of Fig. 2.33, and superior to Fig. 2.32 when apposition is poor.

site system of Figure 2.32. Typically, the plate alone (as in Fig. 2.33) has less than 1% of the rigidity of the bone-plate system acting together.

Of course, the plate may be mounted at right angles to those of Figs. 2.32 and 2.33, in the plane of bending (Fig. 2.34). This arrangement has the advantage that if apposition is poor, the rigidity is much greater—10 to 100 times as great as for the situation in Fig. 2.33. However, the screws are now subjected to bending and torsional forces and these may fail rather than the plate. Also, if apposition is good, this fixation is inferior because the plate is centered at the neutral axis in bending rather than at the extreme fiber, so that total rigidity is less than for the case of Fig. 2.32, and the fracture is not totally in compression. Single plate fixation is thus not recommended when a gap exists at the fracture site. No matter where it is relative to the bending axis, the plate will probably bend or the screws loosen (Fig. 2.35). A comminuted fracture may create the same problem.

Two methods of using two plates to cope with "gaps" are shown in Fig. 2.36. Such fixation is most effective when the axis of the applied moment(s) is well known. In *B*, the two plates suffice to make the fixation act as a composite beam, with one plate in tension and the other in compression, with good rigidity. However, even if not on opposite sides of the bone, two plates provide significantly increased torsional rigidity, as is discussed next.

11. SPIRAL FRACTURES

Section 3 shows that shear stress can result in tensile stresses, which are largest on a plane 45° from the plane of shear. Thus, torsional fractures occur at 45° to the axis of torsion, and the fracture crack, in order to remain at 45° to the applied shear stress, must follow a helical path, that is, it is a "spiral" fracture. In the fixation of such a fracture one must consider this. The forces that tend to disrupt it—the same that tend to disrupt any fracture—are bending and torsion.

If plates are used across the fracture surface but at a 45° angle to the axis of

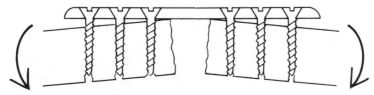

Figure 2.35. Likely consequence of single plate fixation with a gap at the fracture site.

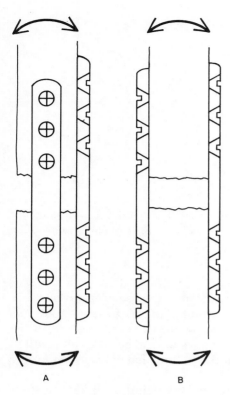

Figure 2.36. Two-plate fixation of gapped or comminuted fractures.

A   B

the bone, as in Fig. 2.37A, the plates resist torsion (on the bone) well, but bending not so well, as shown in Figure 2.37B. In particular, the "tension band" is forced to act at a 45° angle to the extreme fiber stress, which it does not do well. This does not happen if the plate is parallel to the bone; the problems resemble those of Fig. 2.33 in bending! A considerable moment is developed about the screws (Fig. 2.38), however, when torsion is applied.

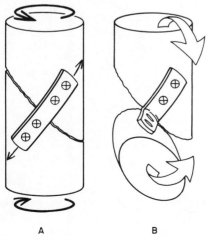

Figure 2.37. Plating across the fracture surface of a spiral fracture resists torsion well *(A)* but bending poorly *(B)*.

A   B

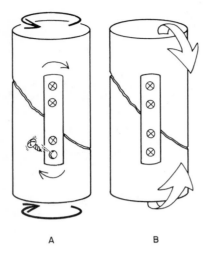

A   B

Figure 2.38. Plating a spiral fracture along the bone axis resists bending reasonably well *(B)* but torsion poorly *(A)*.

A mechanically attractive solution to this problem is the use of straps or wires, as in Fig. 2.39, drawn so tightly as to make rotation of the fragments impossible. This solution is, however, not usually biologically attractive: it can lead to circulatory problems, and in general the high stresses under the wire can result in sufficient resorption to loosen the wires to the extent that there is no longer resistance to torsion.

Two generally viable fixation methods for noncomminuted spiral fractures are shown in Fig. 2.40: a fluted intramedullary rod or a long plate. The flutes in the rod are necessary for torsional stability. The length of the plate serves to reduce the forces corresponding to an applied torque: the moment arms of the forces on the screws are greater, so less force is needed to balance torques and bending moments.

Where plates or rods are undesirable, spiral fractures may be fixed with screws, but with the same problem again: if the screw is placed perpendicular to the fracture surface, optimal torsional stability is obtained, as the screw is parallel

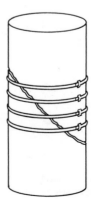

Figure 2.39. Biologically objectionable way to cope with a spiral fracture.

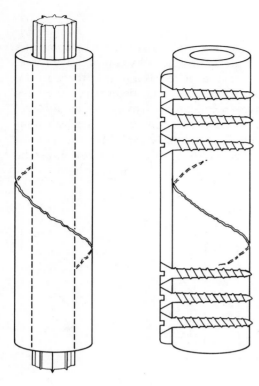

Figure 2.40. Spiral fracture fixed with a fluted intramedullary rod *(left)* or a long plate *(right)*.

to the tensile stress, as discussed above. However, in such a situation, bending moments on the bone cause bending moments on the screw. For optimal bending rigidity the screw should be perpendicular to the axis of the bone, rather than the fracture surface. Where both twisting and bending moments are anticipated (eg, the tibia), one screw may be placed in each orientation, as in Fig. 2.41: now one screw relieves the bending stresses on the other to the same extent, whether the bone is in torsion or bending.

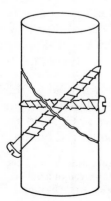

Figure 2.41. Screw fixation of spiral fracture; screws placed to optimize bending and torsional stability.

12. SCREWS

The "tension band" framework includes screws: screws are used to compress fracture fragments together or to hold a plate against bone by compressive force. The balancing force, as in the case of wires and plates, is a tensile force in the fixation device. The screw itself creates such a tensile force, being an elementary machine which is commonly used to convert a small torque to a large axial force. This large mechanical advantage, which makes screws generally useful as fasteners where large holding forces are desired, is particularly useful for the fixation of small fracture fragments. To maximize holding force the screw must be "lagged" as in Fig. 2.42 so that its threads do not separate the fragments.

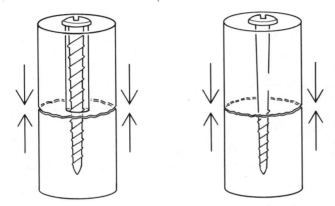

Figure 2.42. Lagging the screw and use of a "lag screw" to assure compression across the fracture surface.

A *"self-tapping" machine screw* with cutters at its tip may be inserted in the drilled hole; or a tool (a "tap") may be used to cut threads in the hole and a machine screw with a smooth end used. To minimize local fracturing and mechanical damage near the screw in bone, the screw hole should be drilled and tapped, ie, threads must be cut in the hole. The cutting edges of the tap are necessarily sharper than the tip of a self-tapping screw, because the tap may be more carefully (and expensively) made, and the tap materials may be high-hardness tool grade alloys which cannot be left in the body due to inadequate corrosion resistance. A sharper cutting edge involves smaller forces and necessarily leaves fewer fragments. A tap cuts cleaner threads than a self-tapping screw and also permits the hole to be flushed of debris before the screw is inserted.

If a single helical thread is cut into a screw, then the pitch (defined as the distance along the screw axis between two parallel loops of the helix) is equal to the lead (the distance the screw advances with each turn) as shown in Fig. 2.43.*

Since pullout of a screw is accomplished by shearing the bone, the holding

---

*A screw (or hole!) may be made with two or more helices, running in parallel, (ie, it may have multiple threads). Multiple-threaded screws advance faster as they are turned: the lead of a double-threaded screw is twice the pitch, so it advances twice as fast as a single-threaded screw having the same pitch.

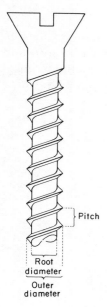

Pitch

Root
diameter

Outer
diameter

Figure 2.43. Descriptive terms for screw threads.

strength of a screw is roughly proportional to the area of a cylinder with length equal to the screw length and diameter equal to the outer diameter of the screw, for the sharp threads shown in Fig. 2.44A.

If the thread shape is bulky or squared, as in the example of the screw in Fig. 2.44B, so that bone is removed from this area by the screw, then holding power is reduced. The thread shape in Fig. 2.44A is much better in this respect. Screws with sharp threads can be used only in pre-tapped holes. Also notice that the thread roots are rounded, to avoid stress concentrations in bending or tension of the screw. This practice greatly enhances the fatigue life of the screw.

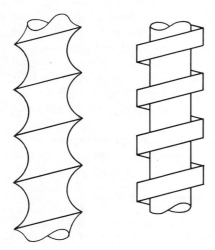

A   B

Figure 2.44. *A*, Thread design with high holding power and fatigue resistance. *B*, Thread design with low holding power.

13. NAILS, RODS, AND PINS

Nails, rods, and pins—in contrast to plates and screws—are intentionally subjected to bending and/or torsion. Consider the femoral neck fracture shown in Fig. 2.45: obviously the force on the femoral head will have a bending moment at the fracture. How large this moment can be may be seen in Fig. 2.46, where

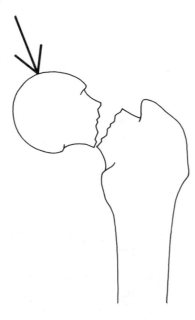

Figure 2.45. The ambulatory force on the femoral head has a bending moment at the fracture site.

the force and moment equilibrium between abductor muscle force and body weight are considered for the left hip when the right foot is off the ground (eg, while walking). We can, in our minds, isolate the rest of the body from the left leg and consider the forces transmitted to the rest of the body from that leg. The forces in this case consist mainly of the abductor muscle force and the hip joint force. The hip joint may be considered as a fulcrum: since the right foot is not on the ground, the abductor muscle acts to keep the trunk level and prevent rotation to the right, by supplying a moment to balance the body weight on the other end of the "lever." However, the lever arm of the abductor muscle is relatively short; typically it is one third of the lever arm of the body weight, with the hip joint as fulcrum. Thus the abductor muscle force may be three times body weight.

Since force equilibrium requires that the hip joint force equals the sum of the muscle force and body weight, the force on the hip joint is four times body weight.* In any case, the joint force indicated in Fig. 2.46 is large—200 to 400

*We have in fact simplified this problem considerably: the weight of the left leg was not subtracted from total body weight; the range of human anatomy contains lever arm ratios larger and smaller than 3:1, and the forces were all assumed to be vertical, whereas the joint force and muscle force are not. A further complication is the presence of dynamic forces, which may considerably exceed the static forces considered here.

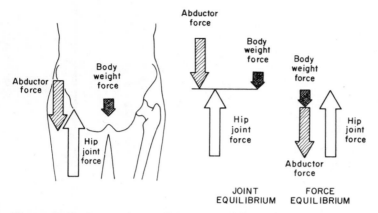

Figure 2.46. Due to its small lever arm about the hip joint, the abductor muscle force must be large to achieve torque equilibrium. The sum of the abductor force and body weight must equal the force on the hip joint to achieve force equilibrium. Thus the force across the hip joint is large, typically four times body weight.

kiloponds (400 to 800 pounds) or more!—and so the femoral neck must withstand a large bending moment when the resultant is not along its axis.

The "tension band" approach would dictate pin placement(s) at point(s) as in Fig. 2.47A which would probably be adequate if in addition to the bending moment there were no *torques* which could cause rotation about the axis of the neck. However, normal walking does cause such torques, and although they are small compared to the bending moment, they are large enough to make fixation with pins (Fig. 2.47A) inadequate with regard to rotational stability (Fig. 2.47B). Thus, if pins are used they must be located as indicated in Fig. 2.48.

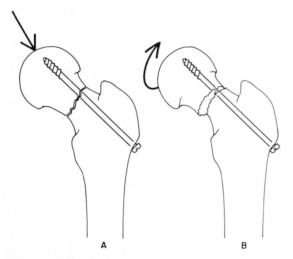

Figure 2.47. Placement of the pin as shown resists the bending moment of the normal joint load (see Fig. 2.46) as shown in *A*; but it does not resist any twisting motions, *B*.

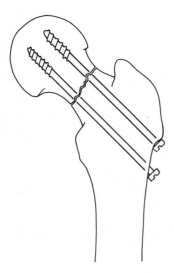

Figure 2.48. Placement of pins to resist joint loading and twisting.

Even so, the static bending forces at the lateral cortex are too high for the bone. This problem may be met by using a nail-plate combination, as in Fig. 2.49. Now, if the bone at the base of the nail resorbs, the bending moment is balanced by forces on the screws in the proximal femoral shaft. Since the screws have reasonably large lever arms, the forces involved are much smaller. These principles are extended further by the arrangement shown in Fig. 2.50, the Deyerle pin and plate device.

The osteotomy compression hook in Fig. 2.51 is more of a "tension band" arrangement than the nail-plate arrangements discussed above. The plate has an external hook to engage the proximal fragment and a cortical screw with an

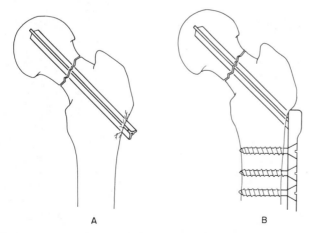

A   B

Figure 2.49. The nail alone results in high forces and possible resorption at the lateral cortex *(A)*; the problem is met by using a plate to transfer and distribute these forces *(B)*; since the lever arm(s) of the screws are great, the forces are lower.

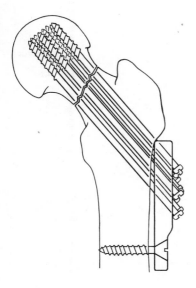

Figure 2.50. Deyerle pin and plate.

eccentric attachment. The fragment is thus compressed against the top of the femur, and the screw assembly is in *tension*.

None of these devices should be expected to bear the normal ambulatory forces by itself; some fail at once at joint forces of 90 kiloponds (180 pounds), when 200 to 400 kiloponds (400 to 800 pounds) are expected (see Fig. 2.46). Thus, bone continuity is essential to successful fixation, as the device must fail if nonunion occurs. For instance, unstable four-part intertrochanteric fractures should be dealt with by stabilizing measures, such as removing bone and placing the head in valgus (Fig. 2.52) or by displacement (Fig. 2.53).

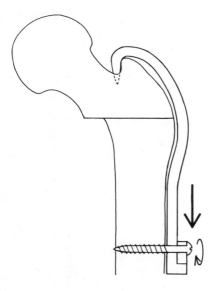

Figure 2.51. Compression hook to fix osteotomies; the hook is in tension, the osteotomy site in compression.

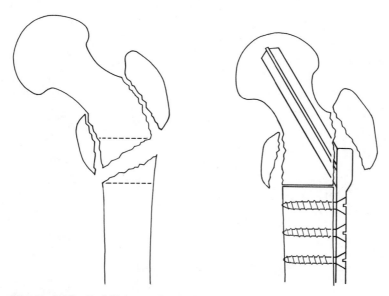

Figure 2.52. Stabilizing a four-piece intertrochanteric fracture. Note that the femoral head is now in valgus.

For simple long bone fractures, intramedullary rods may be used for fixation instead of plates. These fixations are inherently not as rigid as plates since the rod's material is much closer to the neutral axis in bending (and torsion). This may be disadvantageous in certain circumstances; if the bone heals slowly, the rod is more likely to break. On the other hand, the increased flexibility ultimately results in less osteoporosis of the bone near the implant, since the bone must bear

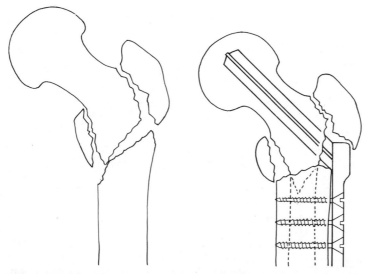

Figure 2.53. Stabilizing a four-piece intertrochanteric fracture by lateral displacement of the proximal fragment.

more of the load. Since intramedullary rods come with a wide range of designs and rigidities, this rationale holds to a lesser or greater degree, depending on the rod design.

The Kuntschner rod, with its cloverleaf cross-section, is relatively strong and relatively resistant to bending because of its considerable area moment of inertia. In other words, it has more material farther away from the neutral axis. However, such a rod design is relatively weak against torsion and a fluted intramedullary rod would be much stronger in this modality (Fig. 2.54).

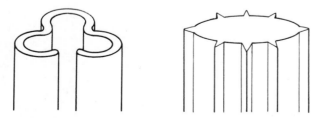

Figure 2.54. The Kuntschner (clover leaf) rod is flexible but relatively weak in torsion compared to a fluted rod.

Intramedullary fixation with a curved rod allows three-point fixation. The rod's concave ends press against the endosteal surfaces of the bone above and below the fracture, and the rod's convex apex presses against the fractured area (Fig. 2.55).

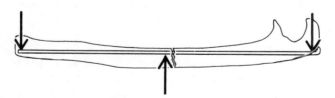

Figure 2.55. Intramedullary rod fixation by three point contact with a precurved rod (or a straight rod in a curved long bone). Flexibility is necessary for such a fixation.

Since long bones naturally curve, it can be argued that straight rods, forced into the medullary cavities, artificially straighten them by angulating the fracture site. The Sage pin was introduced particularly to permit such intramedullary fixation of the radius, the natural curvature of which is essential for full forearm pronation and supination. The Sage pin is relatively flexible and thus weak in torsion, and its use must be augmented by external immobilization. The Rush rod—a small, straight intramedullary rod—has few mechanical advantages. Its use should be confined to bone into small medullary canals, such as the fibula. Rush rods are too rigid to achieve adequate three-point fixation.

Various practical circumstances may dictate the choice of internal fixation devices; comminuted fractures of the long bone, for instance, frequently cannot be reassembled by rods and plates, and screws must be used.

14. BONE GRAFTING

A considerable body of experience indicates that bone grafts have the best results when placed on the tensile side and/or near the neutral axis for bending. The idea is to keep the stress on the bone graft as low as possible, so that it survives and is incorporated. Consider the "prototype long bone," loaded eccentrically as many long bones are, as represented in Fig. 2.56.

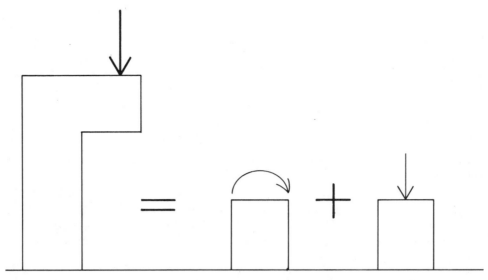

Figure 2.56. "Prototype long bone" loaded eccentrically (off-axis) at the joints. The result is a combination of bending and compressive loading.

Analysis shows that any cross-section has a bending moment and a compressive force on it. The total stress distribution is obtained by simple addition of stresses, as done graphically in Fig. 2.57. The magnitude of the tensile stress at the extreme fiber is less than the magnitude of the compressive stress on the other side, since the stress due to the compressive force cancels some of the stress on the tensile side but adds to the stress on the compressive side. Note also from the figure that the point of zero stress is now no longer at the neutral axis, but nearer to the tensile side. Thus, there is less stress and less movements on the tensile side, which should expedite the establishment of a graft. In this respect, the best location of all is near the neutral axis, but slightly over to the tensile side: the total stress (bending plus compressive load) is zero or nearly so at this location. The bone graft itself does not perform a structural function, but serves rather as a substrata for the growth of new bone.

In cases where a gap is at the fracture site, it is necessary to first stabilize the fracture either with double plates or an intramedullary rod before bone grafting, or otherwise the graft must perform a structural function and will probably fail (Fig. 2.58). An alternative is to bolt double grafts across the gap (Fig. 2.59) but this is generally difficult because the fracture ends are usually osteoporotic and

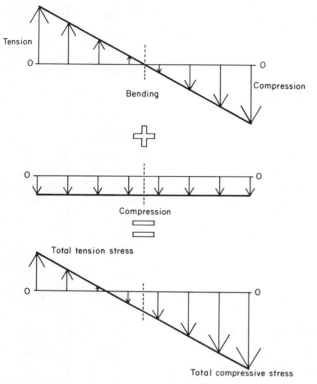

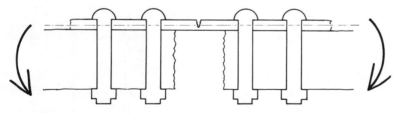

Figure 2.57. Addition of bending and compressive stress patterns across the bone section results in the total stress pattern shown at the bottom. The maximum tensile stress is lowered.

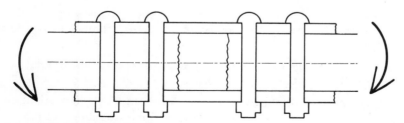

Figure 2.58. Failure of a graft under bending stresses. If a gap exists, the graft must be reinforced by plates or a rod.

Figure 2.59. Double grafts bolted across a gap.

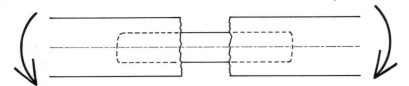

Figure 2.60. Gap bridged with an intramedullary graft.

do not hold bolts well. More practical is the use of an intramedullary fibular graft in the neutral axis, which is thus subject to little stress, while at the same time it acts to stabilize the fracture site (Fig. 2.60).

Eventually, the new bone must grow in response to stress; but the initial graft does best if situated at the point where stresses (and, therefore, strains and relative motion) are lowest.

GLOSSARY

Anisotropic   Directionality of mechanical properties, that is, the material does not behave the same in all directions.

Annealing   Heat treatment used to render metals softer and more ductile.

Anode   In a battery or corrosion situation, the *more* reactive metal which dissolves (ionizes) and gives up electrons.

Area moment of inertia   The relative resistance to bending of a given cross-section. The stress due to bending at any point is proportional to the bending moment and inversely proportional to the area moment of inertia.

Brittle   Sustains little or no permanent deformation prior to fracture.

Casting   Fabrication of parts by melting and pouring into molds.

Cathode   In a battery or corrosion situation, the less reactive metal. It does not corrode.

Center of gravity   Point at which any object is balanced exactly.

Corrosion   Destruction of metal artifacts by electrochemical action.

Ductile   May be deformed permanently without fracture; that is, can be drawn into a wire or rolled into a sheet.

Elastic   Deformation that disappears when the stress is removed.

Elongation at fracture   Permanent (per cent) deformation remaining at fracture; ductile material has a larger elongation at fracture than does brittle material.

Fatigue fracture   Fracture due to repetitive applications of stress not large enough to cause failure with a single application.

Fatigue limit   Repetitive stress that can be endured indefinitely by a particular metal; for stresses below the fatigue limit, fatigue life is infinite.

Forging   Fabrication by mechanical deformation.

Fracture   Failure by the growth of a crack.

Mechanical energy   In the context of this chapter, energy stored in the form of elastic stresses and strains; originally, this energy was work done by applied forces.

Piezoelectric   Solids that respond to applied stresses by becoming electrically polarized. A voltage occurs when forces are applied.

Plastic flow   Deformation caused by shear stress, resulting in permanent changes in shape of any solid.

Polar moment of inertia   Resistance of a given cross-section to twisting; the stress due to twisting (torsion) is proportional to the torque and inversely proportional to the polar moment of inertia.

Self-tapping machine screw   A screw that cuts its own threads in the bone (or other medium) as it turns.

Shear force   Force applied parallel to the surface which tends to either create friction (at the surface) or shear deformation of the interior of the material.

Strain   Percent extension of an object due to the application of stress.

Stress concentration   Point at which the stress is appreciably higher than elsewhere due to geometry of the stressed object.

Surface energy   Energy required to create new surfaces; essentially the energy of broken chemical bonds.

Tensile stress   Tensile (stretching) force divided by the cross-section area.

Tension band   Member that is put in tension in order to compress other portions of the structure (eg, a guy wire).

Torque   Twisting moment.

Toughness   Energy necessary for fracture. A soft, ductile material may be relatively tough.

Ultimate tensile stress   Maximum stress sustainable by a given material.

Yield strength or yield stress   Stress necessary to cause plastic flow.

3
Biomechanics
of Sports Injuries

1. SPORTS INJURIES AND NEWTON'S THIRD LAW

Over the past few years, since statistics on sports-related injuries have been kept, the number of serious musculoskeletal injuries has been increasing. No practicing orthopedic surgeon needs to be told about these statistics: the evidence for this "epidemic" confronts him almost daily in his office. The most dramatic examples are severe cervical spine injuries, particularly from football, rugby, lacrosse, and hockey.

Musculoskeletal elements are torn or broken as a result of high force. In the preceding chapters we discussed force acting on a structure in terms of the stress generated. From a mechanical point of view sports involve the coordinated and skillful manipulation of the body and body segments to achieve a well defined aim, such as to run faster, jump higher, or propel a ball. In all of these activities we either move ourselves or move an object. Now we must consider the rate of travel or speed with which a body segment is moving.

The *momentum* of a moving object, its mass times its velocity, provides tremendous force compared to that generated by the same object when stationary, and accounts for the greater forces associated with collisions of more massive bodies. Velocity is the rate at which an object is moving. Initiating or increasing this rate of motion is *acceleration* which requires energy. To do this we become short of breath and sweat, and our muscles become tired. We're imparting metabolically generated energy to create acceleration, thus transforming *metabolic energy* to energy achieved by the motion of an object, *kinetic energy*. Kinetic energy is quantitatively half the mass of an object times the square of the velocity the mass is moving. Thus kinetic energy is associated with a moving extremity (or anything else!). The faster we accelerate the limb the more *power* (work or energy per unit of time) it possesses. This power allows us to do something with that limb. In all circumstances, the faster the athlete or his body segments are moving, the greater the energy produced.

In sports injuries masses that have achieved considerable momentum as they are powerfully thrust through space collide with other masses, in the form of another player, the ground, the bottom of a swimming pool, or in the case of a moving ball, a glove, bat, or racquet held or attached to a body segment. In any case a rapid, almost instantaneous *deceleration* of some object occurs. Kinetic energy is transferred, dissipated, or converted to other forms of energy. This

90

decrease of the rate of motion of a mass requires just as much energy as did the initial acceleration.

Remembering Newton's third law from Chapter 1, Section 3 (for every action there is an equal and opposite reaction), we can see that what causes injuries in sports is the equal and opposite reaction, either within the limb segment from a collision or from the reaction force created by the acceleration of the body segment itself. For the foot pushing against the ground there is an equal and opposite ground reaction applied to the leg (Fig. 3.1); for the thrown ball there is an equal and opposite reaction applied to the upper extremity.

Reaction force creates kinetic energy within the body segments. The success of the attenuation or dissipation of that energy determines the force and stress levels applied to the anatomic structures. Insufficient shock absorption results in stress concentration and injury.

The effectiveness of shock absorption, the mechanisms by which energy is dissipated, is critical in determining whether or not significant musculoskeletal injury occurs. Consider diving into shallow water and hitting the bottom of the pool (Fig. 3.2).

If the top of your head strikes the unyielding cement floor of the pool, deceleration occurs over a small distance in a short period of time, and fracture-dislocation of the cervical spine almost certainly occurs. However, if kinetic energy built up in the process of diving can be dissipated by the body having sufficient time to decelerate in the water before your head strikes, injury will probably not be severe. If the water is deep enough to allow a more gradual deceleration, so that by the time you get to the bottom little kinetic energy is left, the dive becomes something you can survive. The important concept illustrated here is that gradual deceleration protects because it dissipates much of the kinetic energy; the momentum of the object is slowed gradually.

Having the necessary distance to slow the deceleration process down enough is a way to avoid injury. We *work* to stop the motion. Work is equal to force times

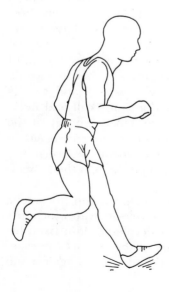

Figure 3.1. As we run the ground imparts an equal and opposite reaction to the foot.

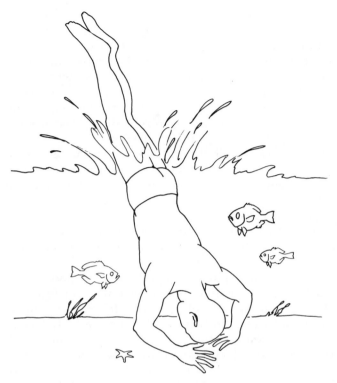

Figure 3.2. Considerable force is generated when the head and hands hit the ungiving surface of the bottom of a pool when one dives into shallow water.

distance. Thus the force related to the work done, or energy required, is inversely related to the distance over which the work is accomplished. The longer the distance over which an object can be decelerated, the less the force required to finally stop it, and thus the less reaction force generated. The extremely short distance for deceleration in the above example therefore implies a large force; hence the spinal damage.

Another mechanism for the gradual dissipation of energy is deformation of surrounding structures. If the pool floor were of thick sponge rubber that would cushion the blow, the deceleration distance would be increased and energy would be used to deform the sponge rubber rather than the skull and neck. Consider the tackling of a charging football player. The kinetic energy of the on-coming player can be substantial (10 to 15 times the energy involved in normal walking) and all of it must be dissipated by forces acting over relatively short distances as the players contact. In head-on tackling (Fig. 3.3) the helmet-protected heads impact with the opposing player.

At first contact the tackled player is traveling at some speed and his kinetic energy is the product of his mass times the square of the velocity with which he's traveling. In order to stop him, another player must decelerate him from his initial velocity to a standstill. This deceleration occurs as the contact force between the helmet and the opposing player builds up and presses against the

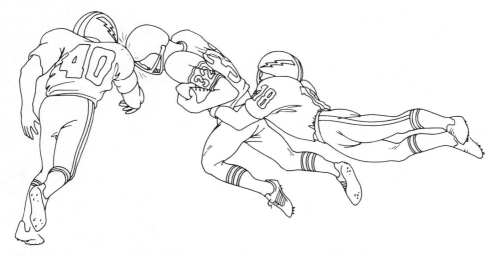

Figure 3.3. In sports related activities such as tackling running players, this rapid deceleration of the runner requires substantial force.

suspension of the helmet and in turn the head of the player acting in the direction opposite the direction of motion of his mass. For the tackler to be decelerated to zero velocity without his gaining much more "yardage," the force times the distance of the decelerating force has to be equal to the initial kinetic energy of the tackler.

In an extreme case if the tackler runs into a rigid stone wall he is stopped but little cushioning is available from the wall and extremely high forces are generated. In the real case, compliance is introduced in several locations, including a falling away of the player being tackled which allows energy to be absorbed over a longer distance, thus reducing the resulting forces. Other cushioning effects come not only from the protective compliance built into the football helmet but also from the compliance of the player's head, neck, other tissues, and bone—and as soon as his shoulder touches the compliance of the shoulder pad of the tackling player. Whether the cervical spine is injured depends crucially on the type of motion allowed when the decelerating force is applied.

Fig. 3.4 generally indicates an impact force on the top of the head centrally in line with the cervical spine. Since the impact force is directed along the axis of the spine, no bending moment is introduced which would tend to flex or extend the spinal axis from its indicated direction. The compliance in this situation arises strictly from the compression of the helmet and its suspension, the skull, vertebral bodies, and discs. Muscles can play only a stabilizing role in this situation since they cannot resist compressive forces.

The loading situation changes significantly when the tackle contact or other impacts to the head are from a nonaxial direction such as a frontal face mask impact or impact from the back of the head causing either extension or flexion of the cervical spine, respectively. In these situations the spine is subjected primarily to a bending mode of loading with general tension generated at the convex surface and compression to the concave surface of the deforming spine. The

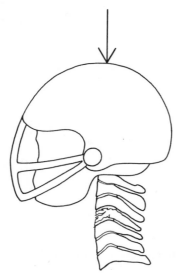

Figure 3.4. Impact loads directly in line with the cervical spine are likely to cause compression fractures.

bending moment acting in any section of the spine is proportional to the moment arm through which the impact forces act. Since the inherent resistance to flexion-extension is rather low, the impact force can travel through a considerable distance before, say, the spinous processes limit further extension and a typical hyperextension fracture of the intervertebral spaces is produced (Fig. 3.5).

In this eccentric loading situation, under certain circumstances, paraspinal cervical soft-tissue muscles can act to reduce the "shock," as is discussed in Section 2.

When impulsive loads to the head tend to bend the cervical spine, the stabilizing ligaments and muscles of the spine can play an extremely important role in absorbing the energy of the impact if considerable deformations can be tolerated. The ligaments and muscle tissue on the tension side of the spine require a

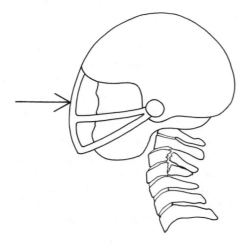

Figure 3.5. Impact loads at some angle to the cervical spine are likely to cause flexion or extension injuries.

stretching force to produce elongation and these forces times their displacement create work at the expense of the impact energy. The tensile force generated in the muscle and connected tendons are transformed into compressive forces in terms of the vertebral bodies and discs. Thus, although the tensile strength of the vertebral bodies is quite low compared to their compressive strength, the geometry of the tendon and muscle containment of the spine together with the available large motions acts to apply compressive rather than tensile force on these skeletal members. Each component of the musculoskeletal system which deforms under the applied load is effectively reducing the energy which has to be dissipated by the remaining components and thus reduces the peak felt by any component of the system.

As the shock or peak dynamic load is created by sudden accelerations or decelerations, the problem of reducing peak accelerations to acceptable levels boils down to increasing the distance over which the energy is dissipated or arranging a more compliant energy reception. When we accelerate our arm to throw or hit a ball after it has been thrown or hit we "follow through" with further arm motion. This dissipates energy and slowly stops the arm. Failure to properly "follow through" can cause injury. Deceleration involves a lowering of velocity with concomitant dissipation of such energy and depends upon the distance over which we can decelerate.

A simpler example which illustrates all of the above is the catching of a powerfully pitched baseball with a catcher's mitt (Fig. 3.6). As the ball strikes the mitt some of the ball's kinetic energy is dissipated by the creation of soundwaves (the pop of the ball hitting the mitt) and in heat and some by deformation of the

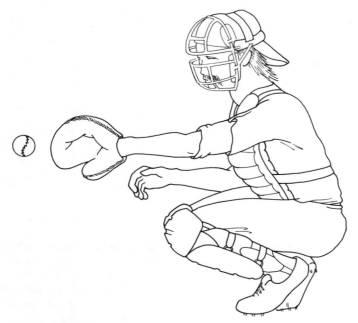

Figure 3.6. Catching a baseball with a catcher's mitt.

material of the mitt itself. But if you hold the mitt steady and unmovable, most of the ball's kinetic energy has to be dissipated over the distance the mitt deforms. Trying to catch a pitched baseball in this fashion results in a bruised palm and possibly even a metacarpal fracture (Fig. 3.7).

Successful catchers decelerate the ball by moving the hand in the same direction the ball is traveling (Fig. 3.8). Thus one can generate the energy required to decelerate and stop the ball with a small force since the force required is multiplied by the distance to achieve the energy transfer. This explains why if you move the mitt back as you catch the ball your hand does not sting. One allows the hand to retract with the ball and decelerate it slowly resulting in small contact forces.

The actual peak force developed during such energy absorption is a direct function of the compliance of the system under the applied load, in other words, how much it moves. Note that under Figs. 3.7 and 3.8 we have plotted the peak forces developed. The area under the curves represents the energy involved, and the area under both curves is equal, because it takes the same amount of energy to stop the ball, whether we bring our glove back or not. That amount of energy is determined by how fast the ball was traveling and its mass. But if we decelerate over a distance we can dissipate the energy with a small force and thus spare the tissues of our hand.

The bony shafts, much as hardwood, bend and deform under applied loads and this bending can act to absorb energy. So can the deformation of the soft

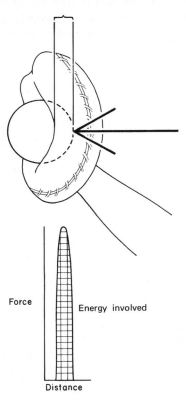

Force

Energy involved

Distance

Figure 3.7. Catching a powerfully thrown baseball in a catcher's mitt without moving the hand decelerates the ball in the distance the glove deforms. This dissipates the kinetic energy of the ball over a relatively short distance, thus generating substantial "peak" force.

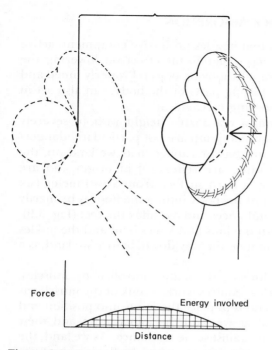

Figure 3.8. Same as Fig. 3.7 except the hand is moved back as the ball is caught. The energy is dissipated over a relatively long distance and the "peak" force developed is substantially reduced.

tissues of the palm. But in catching a powerfully thrown ball with as little contact force as possible, most of the compliance must be produced by muscle action and joint motion which bring the hand and glove back, gradually decelerating the ball.

Enhancing musculoskeletal shock absorption protects athletes from injuries. Helmets that are suspended on the head and allow space in which to deform before crushing into the skull, compliant pads over exposed bony prominences and relatively compliant playing surfaces, and shoes that afford traction but do not rigidly fix the foot on the ground so that the lower extremity can buckle on impact all help.*

Snowmobiles fitted with shock-absorbing seats would probably lower the incidence of compression fractures of the spine which result from the skimobile dropping into ruts and ravines at high speed.

There is no way in contact sports to avoid collision, and it is clearly the unprotected and unprepared for collisions who are injured. Rule changes designed to prevent "blind side" tackles and better designs of protective equipment are goals orthopedic surgeons should promote.

---

*The biomechanical advantage of short skiis with quick release bindings is obvious. While still attached to the foot, skiis act as lever arms multiplying rotational bending forces on the lower extremity. Short skiis decrease this lever arm.

2.   ACTIVE MUSCULOSKELETAL SHOCK ABSORPTION

We have seen in the preceding section that besides protective equipment, active control of limb segment movements has a significant effect on lowering the impact forces felt as we try and stop a rapidly moving object. Properly timed and executed muscle contracture, besides moving parts of the body, can also act in and of itself as a substantial shock absorbing mechanism.

Most of the time we can jump from a reasonable height without severely injuring ourselves. The high jump and broad jump are not particularly dangerous activities. Besides the compliant sand pits or rubber mats we land on, the mechanisms that spare this shock loading are reflexural in origin and are neuromuscular. Most of us can land on a hard surface from a two meter (six foot) height without injury. The impact of the body hitting the floor is primarily absorbed when we straighten the hips and knees and dorsiflex the feet (Fig. 3.9). In order to do this we have to land with the hips and knees bent and the ankles plantar-flexed. Getting them into position on the way down, before we land, is a reflex action.

This extension of the limbs after impact, if totally controlled by muscles, stretches them. The stretching of muscles requires work. Think of the muscles as rubber bands. What the body seems to do is to place the joints into position and by reflex contracts the muscles so that as we land the joints move and their associated muscles are allowed to stretch against some resistance. As we land, the energy of the body hitting the floor is primarily absorbed by flexing the knee and pulling on the contracted hamstrings and gastrocnemius muscles. The "stiffer" the landing, the smaller the deformations and elongations to these muscles, the higher the impact forces.

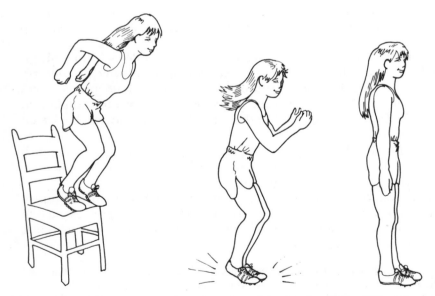

Figure 3.9. We protect ourselves from impulsive loads when we land from a jump by landing with our lower extremities flexed.

When we cannot move and stretch the muscles adequately because we are unprepared for the load, for example as in unexpectedly stepping off a step or when the impulsive load is applied to the long common axis of two limb segments (as if the knee were straight during heel strike), the shock loading has to be completely attenuated or transmitted by the compliance of the loaded skeletal elements themselves: the bone shaft, the cartilage, and whatever soft tissue is in line with these elements. In such a situation muscle cannot contribute substantially to energy reduction because inadequate joint motion is generated to invoke significant reflex action and muscle contraction. In jumping from any height, a stiff-knee landing can be truly painful even from small heights.

Thus controlled joint motion on impact provides several shock-absorbing (energy dissipating) mechanisms. The movement (rotation) of the joint also acts as a dissipater, providing the system with redundant or "wasted" motion. Muscles act to allow the limbs to decclerate over time, lowering the peak dynamic forces generated on deceleration. And finally the active stretching (by segment motion) of muscles under slight tension absorbs vast amounts of energy. One of the secrets of avoiding injuries from impact is to be prepared.

3.   SPORTS INJURY DUE TO FATIGUE

Obviously if the mechanism of skeletal shock absorption by deformation of tissue (and muscular contraction) breaks down due to an abnormal loading situation, or if the total energy of impact exceeds the capabilities of the shock-absorbing mechanisms, fracture of bone and/or rupture of soft tissue results. But damage can result from repeated shock loading, even though each load is well under the threshold the joints and other musculoskeletal tissues can tolerate.

Consider running or hurdling: normally the knee, due to its large range of available flexion-extension and surrounding strong muscles, acts as an extremely good shock absorber because the knee flexes on impact, distributing the required deceleration over a longer distance and absorbing most of the energy by stretching the hamstrings and gastrocnemius muscle (Fig. 3.10). If the runner or hurdler overextends himself, his muscles fatigue and no longer function at just the right moment as to allow them to be stretched under tension. Muscles not contracting at the right moment get overstretched and are strained or sprained. More importantly, the kinetic energy of impact remains to be absorbed to a large extent by deformation of the skeletal tissues themselves. Repeated impact of this nature, although well below the fracture threshold, can produce cumulative damage.

The failure of bone in fatigue is mentioned in Chapter 1, Section 12 and Chapter 2, Section 5. We have also introduced the concept that external loads on the skeletal members are always eccentrically applied, thus primarily creating bending and compressive stresses within the bone and tending to tilt one bone on the other at the joints. Bone is weaker in tension than in compression, and tension is the mode of fracture initiation in bone. Clearly then, lowering the tensile stress minimizes the incidence of fatigue fracture of bone to which the athlete would be particularly prone because of the repetitive nature of sporting activities.

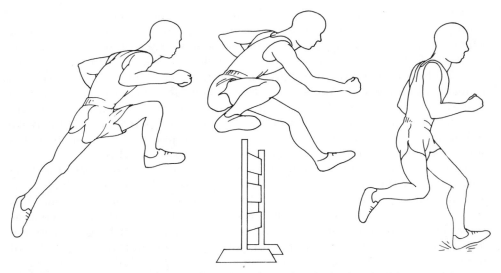

Figure 3.10. Most of the impact from jumping a hurtle is absorbed by stretching the posterior leg muscles.

Experience demonstrates that it is not the well-trained athlete who is subject to the fatigue ("march" or stress) fracture, but rather the "Sunday" athlete. The reason for this is that muscles play a significant role in lowering of the bending stress in bone. Consider the principle of a guy wire used to hold up a radio aerial or telephone pole (Fig. 3.11).

Here the bending stress is lowered and therefore the tensile stresses are significantly reduced (see Fig. 2.57). In a similar manner the iliotibial band lowers the tensile stress in the femur (Fig. 3.12).

The body weight acting centrally tends to bend the femur, creating tensile

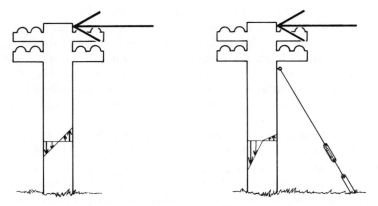

Figure 3.11. The tensile stress created by the attempted bending of a telephone pole can be minimized with a guy wire. Note that the tensile stress is reduced, because the guy wire acts to keep the pole from bending. The guy wire helps pull the pole further into the ground. Thus the compressive stress on the pole is increased.

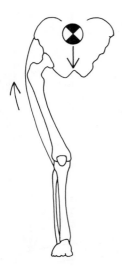

Figure 3.12. The iliotibial band acts as a guy wire, reducing the bending stress on the femoral shaft but increasing its compressive stress.

stress along its lateral edge. The iliotibial band, with its tension controlled by the tensor fascia lata muscle, acts as a tension band and applies a compressive force laterally along the femur, significantly lowering the tensile stresses on that side of the bone. The addition of compressive stress in exchange for a lower tensile stress is a fair trade-off since bone is relatively strong in compression.

Consider the combined effect of the short and long head of the biceps and brachialis in reducing the bending stress in the humerus and forearm (Fig. 3.13A,B,C).

One of the major roles of muscle, besides insuring torque equilibrium and producing motion about joints, is to minimize the tensile stress in bone. Thus fatigue of muscle in the poorly trained athlete creates significant tensile stresses in bone which can result in stress or fatigue fractures. These cracks are essentially an accumulation of fatigue damage at loads below the forces that would normally create fracture.

There is some indication that bone undergoes a continuous process of local damage and rehealing. Because of the nonhomogeneous properties of bone, at a very local level stress concentrations can occur in the bone structure under loads which, although inadequate to damage the overall structure, can produce microfractures. These fractures essentially serve to absorb part of the energy that the overall structure managed to absorb without gross damage, and they relieve the stress on this portion of the overall structure so that continuous application of loads to the overall structure will not lower other portions.

The microfracture, if trabecular, forms a callus which later resorbs, thus healing the local defect. If cortical, the microfracture heals by remodeling. This process appears to be stable at subcritical loads. However, repeated loads exceeding this threshold can produce cumulative microfractures which then accumulate and form stress fractures.

There are also indications that this microfracture mechanism for energy-absorption impact of loading naturally occurs in the subchondral bone of arthordial joints and then an imbalance of the stable equilibrium between micro-

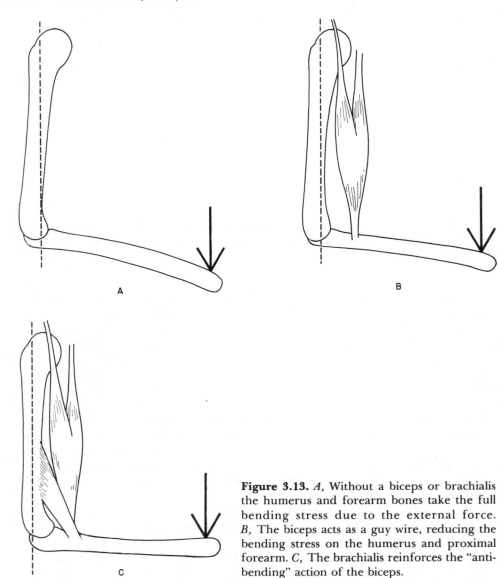

Figure 3.13. *A,* Without a biceps or brachialis the humerus and forearm bones take the full bending stress due to the external force. *B,* The biceps acts as a guy wire, reducing the bending stress on the humerus and proximal forearm. *C,* The brachialis reinforces the "anti-bending" action of the biceps.

fracture and local damage may lead to joint deterioration. Healing of the excessive numbers of microfractures in the subchondral bone can produce local changes in bone stiffness which then create stress concentrations as the load from the cartilage is distributed throughout the subchondral structure. More is said of this in Chapter 4.

4.   MECHANICS OF LOCOMOTION

Most sports involve running. Even in the well trained athlete short bouts of sprinting can be exhausting, whereas walking, for prolonged periods, even in the untrained person, can be accomplished without fatigue. In running we increase our kinetic energy, deriving most of it from an increased metabolism. In walking we minimize the contribution to kinetic energy from metabolic sources. How is this accomplished?

Whenever a mass is elevated, gravity tends to make it fall from its height. Although it takes energy to lift the mass, it falls without the active expenditure of energy, and in fact kinetic energy increases. A mass, which has the potential to fall and thus have gravity act on it, can be considered to have *potential energy,* which is equal to the energy required to lift the mass, and is also equal to the kinetic energy at the end of the fall. In other words, the work done on the mass against the force of gravity is called potential energy. If a person falls, this work is converted to kinetic energy.

Consider a roller coaster (Fig. 3.14). For it to move initially from a stopped position to the top of its track requires acceleration, provided by an engine or motor of some sort. Kinetic energy is expended. As the roller coaster gains altitude it develops potential energy, proportional to the height achieved. At the top of its track it has developed maximal potential energy, and the transfer of kinetic to potential energy is complete. The ride down requires no further kinetic energy. The increased acceleration of the roller coaster on the way down is the result of potential energy; as it gains acceleration, it transfers potential energy to kinetic energy. At the bottom this transfer is complete. In an idealized frictionless environment the roller coaster could just keep on going in the same direction at a constant velocity without the need of additional energy to keep it moving. Frictionless situations never exist on earth and certainly don't exist on roller coaster tracks. In reality one has to apply energy to maintain constant velocity except in outer space.

Potential energy is the quantity of the mass raised multiplied by the height to which it is raised (Fig. 3.15). In discussing changes in the situation of the mass it is easier to think about that mass as if it is concentrated in one point. This point is called the *center of gravity* and it is the spot where one would place a pin in order to balance that mass on the pin. In humans standing at attention the center of gravity is just in front of the second sacral vertebra. With changes in the positions of the limbs and head, as in gait, the center of gravity shifts.

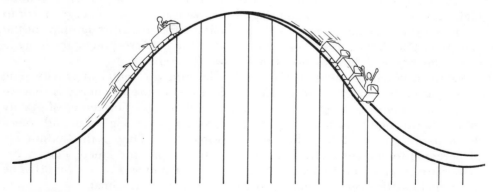

Figure 3.14. A roller coaster requires kinetic energy to get it to the top of its track. The ride down requires no energy—in fact, energy has to be expended to stop it.

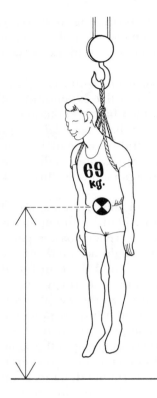

Figure 3.15. Potential energy depends upon the mass of the object and the height to which it has been raised. For convenience, the center of mass (center of gravity) is used for these measurements (see text).

For simplicity of analysis one can describe the motions of the body through space in gait as changes in the position of the center of gravity. A good description of human gait is that we basically elevate our center of gravity, allow it to fall, decelerate it and then accelerate the center of gravity back up. We repeat this process over and over so that we continue walking rather than falling down. Just standing endows the human center of gravity with significant potential energy. To lift the center of gravity up, work is done in addition to the work necessary for forward acceleration (Fig. 3.16).

Potential energy depends on the position of the center of gravity. It is at its highest in the stance phase of gait (Fig. 3.17). We use potential energy in gait to fall forward and achieve a relatively metabolically free ride through part of the gait cycle. The "falling down" part is important as it converts potential energy to kinetic energy, with little or no additional work necessary.

We build potential energy by kinetically elevating the center of gravity. The main reason human gait is so efficient in its expenditure of energy is that we achieve a trade-off between kinetic and potential energy. The center of gravity moves up during the beginning of stance or swing phase (Fig. 3.18) and comes down just after the middle of the stance or swing phase. There is thus a trade-off of potential for kinetic energy in gait. At just the time the kinetic energy demands are greatest, our potential energy is maximal and we can trade it off. The additional kinetic energy demands in gait are therefore minimal.

Kinetic energy is produced by metabolic processes. Most of the metabolic

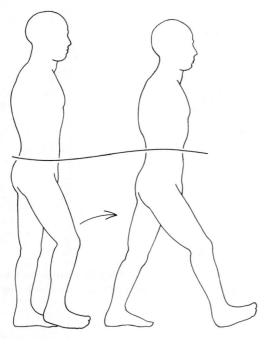

Figure 3.16. As we swing through in gait the movement of the swing leg consumes kinetic energy. Actually most of it is spent decelerating the leg. As a result, kinetic energy is at its peak in the swing phase of gait.

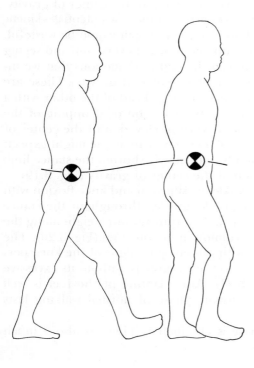

Figure 3.17. As we move over the stance foot we elevate the center of gravity of the body, thus increasing our potential energy. Potential energy is thus greatest in stance, and so can be maximally utilized in the swing phase as the center of gravity drops.

105

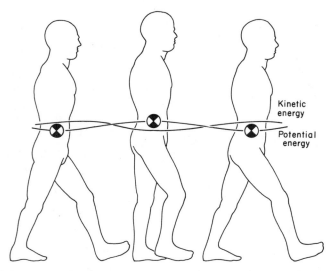

Figure 3.18. Note that in gait, potential energy is maximally available when the demands for kinetic energy are greatest. A trade-off can thus occur, lowering the demands for kinetic energy.

energy expenditure in gait is not used to accelerate the center of gravity but rather to decelerate the inertia created by body motion. Once you "get going" it takes relatively little energy to "keep going."

Clearly we want to minimize energy expenditure, and in forward motion we should not waste energy by an unproductive movement of the center of gravity. Some vertical displacement is of course necessary to achieve a potential—kinetic energy trade-off. But too much up and down motion in gait would be wasteful. The reader can establish this by bouncing up and down at every step and seeing how quickly one tires. There are certain coordinated joint motions that we instinctly use to limit vertical displacements of the center of gravity. These are rotation of the pelvis, which allows us to move one leg ahead of the other with a minimum of excursion of the center of gravity; pelvic tilt or dropping of the pelvis on the swing side which further limits vertical elevation of the center of gravity because it keeps the swing half of the body lower than one might expect; knee flexion on the stance side which tends to relatively shorten the stance limb and prevent unnecessary upward motion of the center of gravity (Fig. 3.19).

The coupling of knee extension with ankle dorsiflexion and knee flexion with plantar flexion, maintains a relatively equal length leg throughout the stance phase as we come down initially on our heel, then transfer our weight along the foot and roll the foot off the ground by coming up on our toes (Fig. 3.20). The relative adduction of the femoral shaft with physiologic valgus of the knee permits the foot to be placed close under the center of gravity without its excessive lateral shift in the stance phase (Fig. 3.21). Also planting of the feet is well coordinated during gait. The double support phase of normal walking lasts about 15% of the gait cycle.

In running the double support phase is eliminated. There is also a much

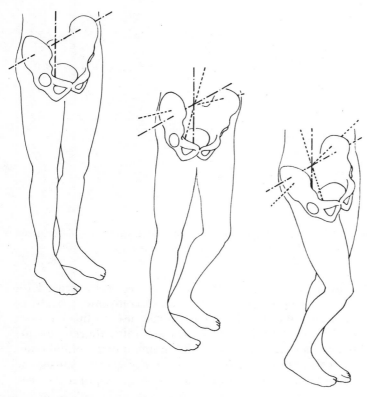

Figure 3.19. Rotation of the pelvis, pelvic tilt, and knee flexion on the stance side all act to minimize excessive vertical motions of the center of gravity during gait.

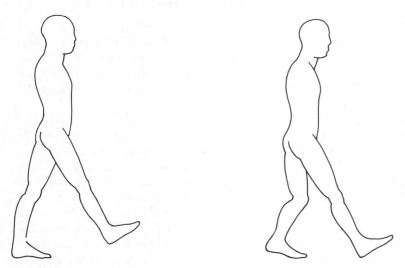

Figure 3.20. Coupling of knee and ankle motions helps maintain a level center of gravity during gait.

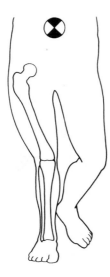

Figure 3.21. Physiologic valgus of the knee minimizes lateral displacement of the center of gravity during gait.

greater vertical displacement of the center of gravity as the legs are used for forward propulsion and there is a substantial upward component of force created in this motion. The lack of a double support phase also requires a wider based foot placement for balance than does walking. In running therefore kinetic energy is increased to such a great extent that the moment of potential energy gained with the larger vertical movements of the center of gravity is insignificant compared to the tremendous amounts of kinetic energy required to keep running.

5.   MECHANICS OF MUSCLE RUPTURE, BURSITIS, TENDONITIS, AND MENISCAL TEAR

In previous sections of this chapter we have stressed how joint motion and muscle lengthening act as shock absorbers and lower the tensile stress on bone. Failures of the muscles and joints in these usually well coordinated activities are not uncommon, and soft-tissue injuries are the most frequent injuries acquired by athletes.

Muscle ruptures if passively pulled beyond its ultimate tensile stress. Given the limitation of joint motion, muscle rupture is usually a rare injury from simple stretch in the absence of direct trauma to the muscles or joint dislocation. More common is complete rupture of a muscle due to forced stretching while it is in contraction. This results from instant incoordination. This is what usually happens when the biceps tendon or heel cord ruptures (Fig. 3.22).

What is more common than complete muscle rupture is partial muscle tear. In the inadequately trained athlete, muscles fatigue. Contractions become insufficient to create the required tension. The athlete keeps trying to perform. Muscle substance is subjected to passive stretch which creates a small, incomplete tear, commonly referred to as a "charley horse."

The tendon sheaths that envelop moving tendons and the bursae that separate

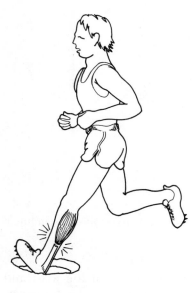

Figure 3.22. Rupture of the heal cord usually results when the gastrocnemius muscle is stretched while it is being forcefully contracted, such as when a runner unexpectantly steps in a hole.

muscles from underlying bony prominences both occur in places where the muscle pull undergoes change in direction and they are subject to trauma at these points. A bursa or tendon sheath is usually located at the fulcrum of a muscle excursion (Fig. 3.23) and in such a place can have considerable compressive force applied to it. Such force can damage the lining of the bursa or tendon sheath, creating inflammation which, if continued, becomes chronic. Such chronic inflammation in a bursa is "bursitis"; in a tendon sheath it is "tendonitis."

Tennis elbow is an excellent example of a chronic tendonitis caused by a

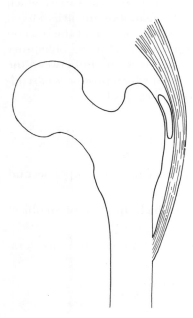

Figure 3.23. Bursas are in areas where a muscle or tendon rides over a bony prominence.

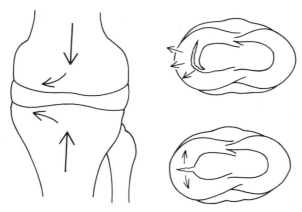

Figure 3.24. Meniscal tears in the knee result from excessive stress on the semilunar cartilages when full knee motion is blocked.

rupture of the deep aspect of the common extensor tendon of the wrist and finger extensors as they originate on the lateral epicondyle of the humerus. Because these extensor tendons are used in almost all hand motions, this area is almost never rested and the sprain becomes associated with inflammation and remains chronic. Attempts to treat tennis elbow mechanically by taking the strain off the extensor tendons with a tight upper forearm band, or with a larger grip racquet handle or a change in stroke, particularly in the back hand, are usually successful.

The most common serious sports related soft-tissue injury is a tear of the semilunar cartilage or meniscus of the knee. Such injuries normally result from a blow to the knee in a situation which fails to allow adequate knee motion to dissipate the energy. This results in extremely high intra-articular forces which exceed the tensile strength of a semilunar cartilage. Knee motion involves a fixed coupling of a flexion-extension with internal and external rotation of the tibia on the femur. If the knee is flexed or extended in such a way that the obligatory concomitant rotation cannot be carried out, the meniscus is caught between the tibial condyle and the femur under a shearing type load which produces extruding type stress with tension in the direction shown in Fig. 3.24.

GLOSSARY

Acceleration   Rate of increase of an object's velocity (meters or feet per second per second).

Center of gravity   For analytical purposes, point at which the mass of an object can be thought to be concentrated.

Deceleration   Rate at which a moving object is slowed (same units as acceleration).

Inertia   Tendency of a mass to resist changing velocity.

Kinetic energy   Energy achieved by the motion of an object, determined by multiplying half the mass times the square of the velocity the object is moving.

Metabolic energy   Processes by which a living organism creates energy from its food.

Momentum   Mass of the object multipled by its velocity.

Potential energy   Energy due to work done against the force of gravity, that is, an increase in the height of the center of mass.

Power   Work or energy per unit of time.

Work   Force times distance.

4
Mechanics of Joint Degeneration

1. OSTEOARTHROSIS AS A WEAR AND TEAR PHENOMENON

Although metabolic and enzymatic factors are involved in joint degeneration (osteoarthrosis), the process is best thought of as the final common pathway of mechanical deterioration of joints, occurring from an imbalance between the stresses applied to the joint and the ability of the tissues to resist that stress. Thus osteoarthrosis can result from either excessive or poorly handled stress or from an inherent structural weakness of the articular cartilage. In the latter situation the mechanical implications are clear. The yield stress of the cartilage is lowered and even normal stress overwhelms its structural integrity.

In this biomechanical approach we will not discuss joint degeneration associated with underlying metabolic abnormalities and discuss only situations clearly associated with a primary mechanical cause. Incongruity, from any cause, results in stress concentrations within a joint. So does relatively unprotected trauma. If the traumatic forces are severe enough, fracture of a long bone or rupture of ligaments results. Low level, repetitive trauma is most likely to cause osteoarthrosis. For example, pitching a curve in baseball involves a rapid rotatory acceleration or snap of the forearm when the ball is released. The elbow joint lacks effective shock absorbing mechanisms to protect the radiocapitellar articular cartilage from such a repetitive insult and osteoarthrosis results. This can occur even in skeletally immature persons and has been the reason behind attempts to ban the curve ball from "Little League" competition.

It is not unusual for the stress on articular cartilage to be 1.4×10^6 to 3.5×10^6 newtons per square meter (200 to 500 pounds per square inch). Even under such punishing repetitive loading, most joints function well for decades. This chapter discusses how joints mechanically function and the role mechanical factors can play in the development and treatment of osteoarthrosis.

2. STRESS DISTRIBUTION WITHIN JOINTS

The load across the joint is the (vectorial) summation of (1) body weight plus the forces due to acceleration and deceleration of the segment and (2) the muscular forces required to stabilize the joint and move the limb. The contribution from the muscular forces in most cases provides the bulk of the overall force across the joint (see Fig. 2.46). In order to minimize the stress across the joint this load is distributed over a contact area that is substantially greater than that of the bony shafts, creating the familiar bulbous ending of the bones at their articulations.

The bearing surface of joints consists of two thin layers of cartilage separated by an extremely thin layer of synovial fluid. The cartilage sits on two relatively thick pads of cancellous bone. To minimize the stress on the cartilage it is desirable to distribute the load over as large a contact area as possible. As the joint is loaded, the cartilage and bone deform. Although the cartilage is about 10 times more compliant (less stiff) than the underlying cancellous bone, the cartilage is relatively thin, and thus its total actual deformation is limited. The cancellous subchondral bone, although stiffer, is of sufficient depth to permit significant total deformation and thus allow the joint to maximally conform under load, creating the largest possible load-bearing contact area (Fig. 4.1).

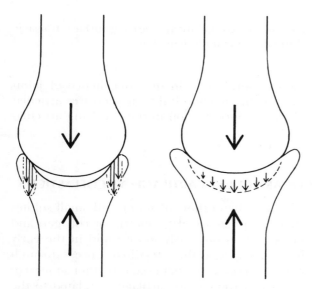

Figure 4.1. Under load the joint conforms, to some extent, through the deformation of cartilage, but under high loads mostly by local deformation of the subchondral cancellous bone. Note what happens to the stress distribution if joint conformation does not occur.

Cartilage acts mainly as a bearing surface and transmits the stress applied to it to the underlying bony bed (Fig. 4.2). The subchondral cancellous bone of the metaphysis then acts in two ways: first, by deformation of the bone the joint achieves a maximum contact surface and thus a maximum load-bearing area under high loads; secondly, the cancellous bone is arranged in trajectories which transmit the major part of the stress down onto the shaft (Fig. 4.3).

Trabecular bone deformation also provides some minor shock absorption and thus acts to absorb energy. Trabecular microfracture naturally occurs. This energy of fracture is thus absorbed by the bone tissue. As long as the frequency of these microfractures is low compared with the rate of healing, significant alterations in the deformability of the cancellous bone is not evident. However,

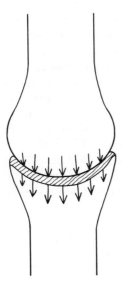

Figure 4.2. Cartilage acts mainly as a bearing surface, transmitting applied forces to the underlying bone.

because of the importance of subchondral bone in the congruence of joints under load, loss of the compliance of the subchondral bone increases articular stress and can lead to high local stress concentration in the overlying articular cartilage (Fig. 4.1).

3. MECHANICAL BEHAVIOR OF ARTICULAR CARTILAGE: VISCOELASTICITY

Under load, articular cartilage deforms by outflow of water and small solutes which are trapped by the highly hydrophilic cartilage matrix of collagen and proteoglycan. The rate of water outflow is obviously more rapid in the early stages of deformation than in the later stages, as the interstitial "pores" through which this flow takes place become narrower as the material is further squeezed. Since the deformation of a fully soaked sponge, as cartilage, is related to the amount of trapped water that has run out, squeezing with a constant load results

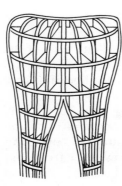

Figure 4.3. Schematic representation of the cancellous structure of metaphyseal bone. The longitudinal plates of bone act to transmit the joint stress down onto the diaphyseal shaft. These longitudinal plates are reinforced by transverse interconnecting plates or struts.

in a nonlinear deformation. Initially water comes out easily and it deforms rapidly. The more the cartilage is wrung out the more difficult it is to get the last bit of water out.

The second unique behavioral characteristic of such a system is that the deformation is closely related to the rate at which the external force is applied. The faster it is squeezed, the harder it is for the water to come out; the more slowly it is squeezed, the easier it is to get all the water out. Such rate dependence of deformation is different from the deformation of common engineering solids. Materials such as wood and metal deform a given amount for a given amount of stress in a linear fashion, elastically. Cartilage deformation is nonlinear as it depends upon fluid flow and this strain rate dependent deformation is called *viscoelastic*. (Bone under some conditions has viscoelastic properties as well.)

The hydrophilic matrix of cartilage tends to maintain water within its substance, creating pressures within it. This pressurized liquid can carry load as can the pressurized abdominal contents described in Chapter 1, Section 8. As discussed there, the carrying of load by such equilibrated pressurization is called hydrostatic pressure, and has a high compressive yield stress.

4. MECHANICAL FACTORS IN THE WEARING AWAY OF ARTICULAR CARTILAGE

Although chemical, enzymatic, and metabolic factors can lower the yield strength of articular cartilage, the wearing away of the bearing surface down to bare bone requires mechanical forces. Termites can weaken a piece of wood, but the wood never breaks up into pieces unless it is subjected to some sort of a loading stress.

From a mechanical point of view, one may separate cartilage fibrillation initiation, propagation, and loss of substance. Cracks and tears beginning in the surface tangential fiber layer must, by definition, be initiated by tensile stress, that is, a pulling of the structure apart. As is discussed in Section 6, joints are lubricated so well that shear forces at the articulating surfaces at best play only a secondary role in cartilage wear. The major loads across the joint are compressive in nature. How then are tensile stresses produced?

If articular cartilage were compressed evenly across its entire surface no tensile stresses would exist. In whole joints however this is probably never the case. Only a part of the joint surfaces is load-bearing at any instant. Since adjacent areas of the cartilage surface are connected, if one area is compressed and another is not, the tissue connecting them is stretched in tension. In this way tensile stresses occur at the periphery of loaded areas (Fig. 4.4).

Articular cartilage is designed so that it has maximal resistance to being broken apart. The fiber phase of articular cartilage is collagen. Its general arrangement (unloaded and loaded) is shown in Fig. 4.5. At the surface it is arranged to resist tensile stresses by being oriented tangential to the surface. Despite this, it can fail under repetitive normal loads, which accounts for the almost universal findings of fibrillation around the periphery of joints in older persons (see Fig. 4.4).

The propagation of cracks in cartilage depends upon the same factors as does

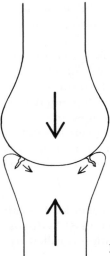

Figure 4.4. Tensile stresses occur in articular cartilage at the margins of the contact zone. Fibrillation initiates there.

their initiation. An increase in the length of a fibrillation (crack) or ultimately even the possible tearing away of an area of cartilage from the calcified bed must involve the generation of tensile stresses. Local stresses within cartilage are dependent on the applied stress, Young's (elastic) modulus of the fibrillated cartilage, Young's modulus of the bony bed, and the stress gradient between adjacent areas of subchondral bone.

The midzone fibers of collagen, although randomly oriented in position in the unloaded state, under compression line up in an optimum configuration along

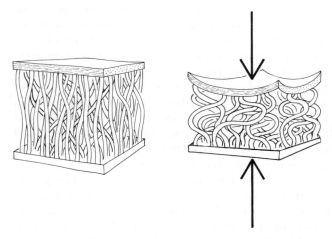

Figure 4.5. Schematic representation of cartilage collagen. The fibers are not really that long. Unloaded, their orientation in the central zone is fairly random. Upon compression the predominant orientation in the middle zone becomes perpendicular to the load.

tensile lines to resist crack propagation. If enzymatic degradation or cellular metabolism has weakened this structure, normal levels of repetitive stress could create failure conditions. If this has not occurred, high stress levels must be present to propagate a crack. Such high local tensile stress concentrations can occur where the compressive stresses created in the cartilage are uneven. Such a situation arises when cartilage has structural or geometric alterations secondary to inherited or developmental abnormalities or attempts at cartilage repair.

Uneven compressive stresses in the cartilage may not only arise from irregularities within its own structure, but from uneven stresses in the underlying subchondral bone in continuity with the cartilage. Normal joint structure, even in its deepest layers, is designed to prevent any sharp stress gradients. At the junction between relatively deformable articular cartilage and stiff cancellous bone is an intervening layer of calcified cartilage of intermediate Young's modulus, which assists in the smooth transmission of stresses. The deepest zone of collagen fibers cross these layers and act as an anchor. Furthermore, the junction between cartilage and its calcified bed is not straight but undulates. This increases the surface area and maximizes the possibility of transmitting compressive stresses rather than tensile stress, from shear.

Despite this, steep gradients between adjacent sections transversely across the joint can occur in the deep layer from the natural loading patterns in certain joints (Fig. 4.6). For example, such an area is in the medial central facet of the patella, a common site for cartilage fibrillation. Such local steep stiffness gradients can also occur from alterations in the stiffness of the subchondral scleroses secondary to intra-articular fractures. Multiple repetitive impulsive loads, poorly handled by the musculoskeletal shock absorbers (see Chapter 3) can so stiffen subchondral areas of bone.

Although local stiffness gradients can be associated with cartilage fibrillation, the progression of this fibrillation to total loss of cartilage substance down to bare bone appears to be related to the relative stiffness of its underlying cancellous bone. Osteoporotic, relatively compliant bone appears to spare its overlying cartilage from severe mechanical deterioration, probably because on such a compliant bed sufficient shear stresses in the cartilage depths cannot be generated. (It is easier to abrade tape off a hard surface than off a sponge.) As Newton's first law has taught us, the shear force generated cannot exceed the capacity of the tissues to provide an equal and opposite force.

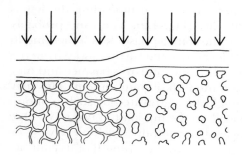

Figure 4.6. Sharp gradients in the stiffness of the underlying subchondral bone create tensile stress in the cartilage overlying the gradient and can lead to cartilage fibrillation in this area.

5.   MECHANICAL CONSIDERATIONS IN THE TREATMENT OF OSTEOARTHROSIS

Cartilage "wear" results when the ultimate tensile strength of cartilage is exceeded. However, contrary to popular teaching, once this process is started, it is not always irreversible. There are well recorded instances of clinical remission of osteoarthrotic joints, and remission has been achieved clinically and experimentally and by surgical intervention. All the metabolic evidence accumulated to date suggests that the joint is capable of healing response. Failure to heal may be due to a persistent "relatively" high level of stress in the joint. If these stresses can be sufficiently lowered, one can expect some functional healing of both bone and bearing surface to take place.

Stress in a joint can be diminished in one of two ways: the overall load on the joint is decreased or the surface area over which that load acts is increased.

Decreasing the Overall Load on the Joint

The use of external aids to ambulation (walker, crutches, or cane) throughout the world is the most common form of treatment of osteoarthrosis. Of these aids, a walker most disrupts the normal gait cycle. It must be picked up and moved at each step which interrupts the normal rhythm of gait and denies the use of momentum as an energy-saving device. It is popular with older persons because it significantly enlarges their base of support and does not require significant shoulder and upper upper arm muscles. In actuality the walker is the external aid of choice for patients with a low energy reserve.

Bilateral crutches allow the shoulder muscles to be used effectively and permit some momentum to be applied in the gait cycle. Crutches are most effective when used in combination with a partial weight-bearing gait so that the weight of the limb is rested on the ground, making it unnecessary for the person to totally support the limb in the stance phase (Fig. 4.7). Under such circumstances crutches can free the lower extremity of almost all its load by mainly making it unnecessary to contract the muscles in order to stabilize the hip or leg. Contrary to intuition, a nonweight–bearing crutch gait loads the joints of the lower extremity more than does a touch-down gait because the muscles must contract to carry the weight of the leg (Fig. 4.8). Theoretically this gait takes about 80% of the load off the joints in the stance phase in that leg, as compared to 90 to 95% reduction with a touch-down gait.

In a similar manner, a cane obviates the need for the abductors of the hip on the affected side to contract but is much less effective in unloading the leg as muscles still have to contract for some stability (Fig. 4.9). The cane probably relieves about 60% of the load on the hip in the stance phase. It is something to lean on for support and will have its longest lever arm the further away from the affected leg the tip of the cane is put down. The cane improves balance and may allow the leg to be brought through with a minimum of joint motion. This may spare inflamed areas of synovium which might be aggravated by such motion.

One can surgically decrease the overall load on the hip joint in two ways. One method consists of lengthening the muscles by tenotomy, such as a Voss or "hanging hip procedure." The length of a muscle and the strength of its contrac-

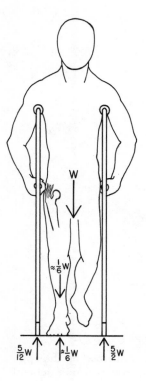

Figure 4.7. The effect of a "touch-down" crutch gait is to eliminate almost all the joint loads in the lower extremity by making it unnecessary for the muscles to stabilize the leg. Since the normal joint forces in the lower extremity are several multiples of body weight (w) the residual weight of the leg (about ⅙w) can almost be ignored.

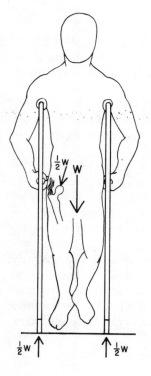

Figure 4.8. A non–weight bearing gait requires muscle contraction to balanced against body weight, such a gait is not as load restrictive as a touch-down gait (see Fig. 4.7).

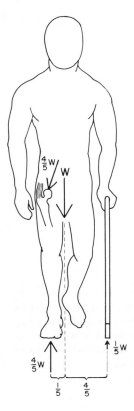

Figure 4.9. A cane theoretically reduces the load on the opposite leg by about 60%. The amount of load reduction depends on how far away from the body the cane is held.

tion are directly related, and when these tenotomized muscles heal with segmental noncontractile elements in series (Fig. 4.10) they are lengthened and their strength is at least one grade weaker than before. A considerable proportion of contraction is dissipated in the scar.

This multiple tenotomy method decreases the overall force, at least transiently, and may provide sufficient time for the joints to heal. Over time the muscles adjust to their new resting length and in some instances regain their initial strength or close to it.

The other method of decreasing the overall load on a joint is by increasing the moment arm of a muscle so that less force is needed to produce a given torque. Around the hip this can be done with a varus osteotomy (Fig. 4.11). In such an osteotomy the lever arm of the femoral neck is lengthened, thus increasing the lever arm of abductors. These balance the forces eccentrically exerted on the hip by the *partial body mass.**

As discussed in Chapter 2 the abductors act through a lever arm which is only a third of the lever arm of the forces exerted by the body mass. Therefore to insure moment equilibrium they must develop a force of about three times that exerted to the body mass, and the total load supported by the joint approximates about four times the body weight. Lengthening the lever arm of the abductor

*This is, of course, the mass of the body minus the leg below the joint being discussed.

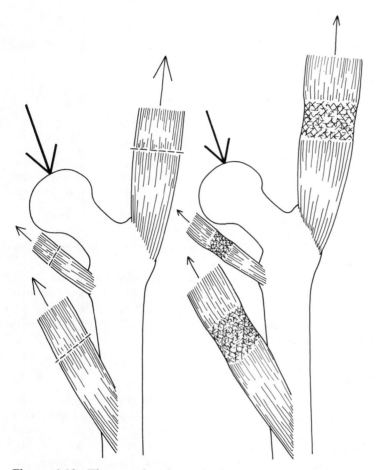

Figure 4.10. The muscles about the hip can be surgically lengthened, reducing their force of contracture, at least temporarily, by about 20%.

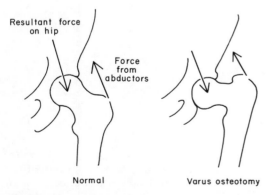

Resultant force on hip

Force from abductors

Normal   Varus osteotomy

Figure 4.11. A varus osteotomy increases the lever arm of the abductors and thus decreases the force required by these muscles to produce a given torque.

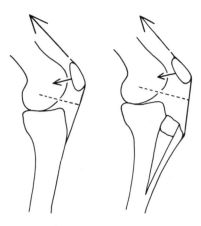

Figure 4.12. The lever arm of the quadriceps can be increased by anterior displacement of the tibial tubercle.

muscles allows them to achieve equilibrium with a smaller force and hence reduces the overall load on the hip joint (see Fig. 2.46).

The principle of decreasing force by lengthening the lever arm is universal and can be applied to any joint where it is surgically feasible. The compressive force exerted by the patella against the femoral groove can be decreased by lengthening the lever arm of the patellar tendon. This can be achieved by displacing the tibial tubercle anteriorly (Fig. 4.12).

Increasing the Weight-Bearing Area of the Joint

The stress in a joint can be decreased by increasing its load-bearing area. The most obvious example is valgus osteotomy in a varus deformity of the knee. With a varus deformity most of the load is transmitted through just one compartment of the knee. After osteotomy it is evenly distributed (Fig. 4.13). Proper corrective osteotomy allows both medial and lateral compartments to bear equal load. Osteotomy is a well recognized and accepted measure for treating osteoarthrosis of the knee which is associated with an angular deformity.

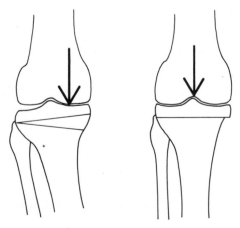

Figure 4.13. With a varus deformity of the knee most of the load is transmitted through the medial compartment. After valgus osteotomy the load is distributed more evenly.

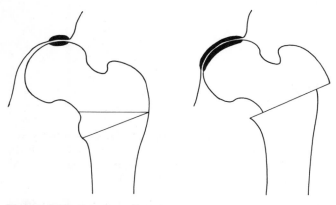

Figure 4.14. In cases of osteoarthrosis of the hip, where congruity is maintained, varus osteotomy may increase the load-bearing surface of the hip while it decreases the overall load (see Fig. 4.11).

Osteotomy about the hip increases the load-bearing area of that joint in certain cases. Generally where congruity is good, especially abduction of the leg, a varus osteotomy is indicated (Fig. 4.14). In cases where a large medial osteophyte has laterally subluxed the hip, for example in an old congenital dysplasia, a valgus osteotomy can bring the osteophyte into the load-bearing area, significantly increasing it (Fig. 4.15). Valgus osteotomy does not move the resultant force on the hip lateral to the acetabulum and thus has no tendency to cause further subluxation.

Valgus osteotomy, however, does decrease the lever arm of the abductors, compelling them to increase their strength of contraction to achieve a torque equilibrium about the hip. This increases the overall load on the hip (Fig. 4.16).

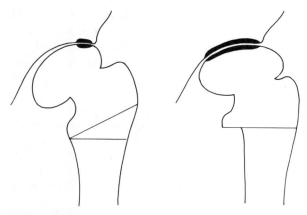

Figure 4.15. In cases of osteoarthrosis of the hip, with a large medial osteophyte, valgus osteotomy can bring that osteophyte into the load-bearing area significantly increasing the contact area. Since valgus osteotomy increases the force on the hip by decreasing the lever arm of the abductors, concomitant procedures must be done if the stress on the hip is to be significantly decreased.

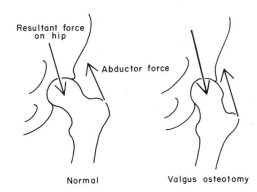

Figure 4.16. A valgus osteotomy decreases the lever arm through which the abductor functions, increasing the overall load across the hip joint.

For this reason a valgus osteotomy must be carried out in conjunction with a hanging hip or Voss procedure, or else the stress on the joint is not lowered, even though its load-bearing surface is increased.

Mechanical Stimulation of Fibrocartilaginous Healing

Fibrocartilaginous healing of areas of destroyed articular cartilage requires a source of cells (usually present either in subchondral bone or in surrounding soft tissue), decreased stress, and motion. Active motion or active assisted motion contracts muscles across the joint and increases the stress. Therefore, for the first several months after osteotomy, active motion should be kept to a minimum.

It has been shown experimentally that primitive pleomorphic fibroblasts, subjected to equal pressure from all directions, produce fibrocartilage (see Fig. 2.27). Continued motion of the healing joint provokes the formation of synovial fluid and creates stresses in the healing mantle over the articular surfaces. If these surfaces are relatively congruent, and the stresses are not excessive, the pressurized synovial fluid transmits hydrostatic pressure. This tends to promote differentiation of chondroid material. Motion apparently orients the superficial fibers of the healing fibrocartilage tangential to the surface and those fibers next to the bone perpendicular to the surface. Over time, maturation of the chondroid bearing surfaces gives a hyaline appearance to the tissue. Too high a stress in the initial healing periods probably increases the tensile stresses to such an extent that the healing surface tissue is ripped apart.

The unreliability of interposition arthroplasty of the hip probably relates to the fact that the surgery and postoperative course do not adequately provide the significant lowering of stress for a sufficient period of time. There is also a question raised by some that such an extensive procedure creates osteonecrosis under the metal mold, but most carefully examined specimens suggest the failures were due to stress concentration rather than to primary vascular insufficiency.

6.   FRICTION ACROSS JOINTS

Joint lubrication is discussed at the end of this chapter because failure of lubrication mechanisms is not believed to be primarily responsible in most clinical situations for joint degeneration. Nevertheless the subject of joint lubrication is important for a complete understanding of joint mechanics and has significant implications in the functioning of total joint replacements, the subject of Chapter 5.

Joints function as the articulations of the skeletal system and must provide relative motion of the body segments while transmitting load. Theoretically then, during articulation, shear forces arise at the interface of the articulating surfaces, and these shear forces have to be overcome by muscle action to produce motion. Synovial joints undergo a variety of loading and motion conditions during normal activity. These range from relatively low to high loads and with a varying velocity of sliding of the opposing cartilage surfaces. Loading can be intermittent and is often impulsive. Therefore, joints must be lubricated by a mechanism that functions effectively for all types of conditions or by several different lubricating mechanisms in order to insure low friction under the full range of operating conditions.

The frictional resistance developed between the articular cartilage surfaces in a joint depends on how much the surfaces actually touch. The less they touch, the easier the two surfaces slide. Obviously the amount of force tending to drive one surface into another, that is, the load applied across the bearing, has an effect on how easy it is to push or pull one surface over the other.

The constant that relates load and frictional resistance is the *coefficient of friction*. It is obtained by dividing the load (kiloponds or pounds) into the force of frictional resistance (kiloponds or pounds). Thus the coefficient of friction is a unitless measure by which the frictional resistance of various bearings can be compared. It is independent of the amount of surface areas in contact with each other. Examples of approximate coefficients of friction are: a steel-on-steel bearing lubricated by oil, 0.210; a plastic-on-metal total hip replacement lubricated by synovial fluid, 0.060; an ice skate on ice lubricated by water, 0.030; and articular cartilage on articular cartilage lubricated by synovial fluid, 0.002. These numbers show that a synovial joint is 100 times easier to move than a steel-on-steel bearing and about 30 times easier to move than a plastic-on-metal total hip replacement.

Note that in the above examples the lubricant is always specified. Lubricants act to keep the surfaces apart thus decreasing the shear forces acting between them. A well oiled bearing moves more easily than a dry one. As the friction developed is the resistance to shear, in most cases it is much easier to shear a fluid lubricant than a solid surface. A property of a well lubricated system is that under the conditions of load which are applied the lubricant is always present and is not squeezed out of the bearing interface or else its effect is diminished.

Two major mechanisms function at the cartilage interface to maintain lubrication, either or both acting according to the load and motion conditions in the joint at a particular time. At one extreme is a *boundary lubrication* phenomenon. Here molecules from the synovial fluid attach themselves by chemical interaction to the articular surfaces.* These bound molecules create a boundary layer which when rubbed against itself offers less resistance to shear forces than would rub-

---

*The boundary lubricating molecules for synovial fluid are a moderate size glycoprotein, chemically distinct from hyaluronate. The role of hyaluronate in joint lubrication is discussed later in this section.

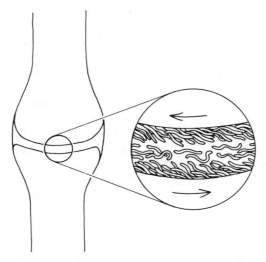

Figure 4.17. Boundary lubrication involves the binding of lubricating molecules to the bearing surface.

bing the two bare articular surfaces against each other (Fig. 4.17). This situation may be likened to a wax coating on the floor or teflon on a frying pan, and is one of the many reasons why such surfaces are slippery. In joints the boundary layer does not operate at high loads as it is too fragile to withstand the shear forces created under such conditions.

How then may a lubricant be kept in an oscillating bearing under high loads and speeds? Several possibilities exist. In most bearings the lubricant is held in place by the physical force generated by the relative sliding motion of the bearing pushing the lubricant ahead. This mechanism is called *hydrodynamic lubrication* and depends upon the relative motion of the opposing surfaces to maintain the wedge of fluid lubricant (Fig. 4.18).

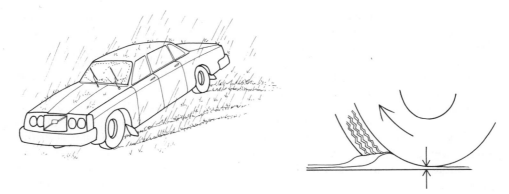

Figure 4.18. Hydrodynamic lubrication involves the maintenance of a fluid between the bearing surfaces due to the relative motion of the bearing. A wedge of lubricant forms at the leading edge of bearing contact. An automobile skids on a wet road due to loss of friction caused by a hydrodynamic phenomenon.

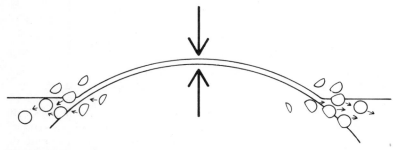

Figure 4.19. Weeping lubrication results when fluid is pushed up into the joint space at the periphery of the zone of impending contact.

Hydrodynamic lubrication is unsuited for diarthrodial joints because a lubricating wedge of fluid cannot be maintained in an oscillating bearing. In such bearings, as a wedge of fluid is built up it is quickly destroyed by the rapid reversal in direction of motion of the bearings.

In joints the lubricating mechanism that appears to be present under high loads and speeds is based on a self pressurized hydrostatic phenomenon called *weeping lubrication*. Instead of the fluid being pushed forward into the contacting space from behind it is pushed up from within the substance of the contacting surfaces themselves (Fig. 4.19). As the joint is loaded the lubricant in the zone of potential contact is pressurized and with cartilage deformation the interstitial fluid from the cartilage is squeezed out of the cartilage around the periphery of impending contact area.*

As the joint slides, the wept fluid is caught between the lubricating parts and adds a low viscosity component to the synovial fluid already trapped in the area, aiding in the separation of the cartilage surfaces. Pressurized fluid or hydrostatic lubrication is an effective way of maintaining fluid and position against an external force. In industry, pumps are used to maintain hydrostatic pressure. In joints, the articular cartilage under load self-generates pressure which squeezes the fluid in the cartilage out.

Thus the relative sliding motion of the joint accompanied by compression of the cartilage results in the pressurized fluid film between the surfaces composed of entrapped synovial fluid and wept cartilage interstitial fluid (Fig. 4.20). This hydrostatic self-pressurized lubrication is most effective in high loads and particularly during transient or impulsive loads.

The relative sliding motion of two compliant surfaces over each other allows some deformation horizontally and may aid in lowering the frictional resistance (Fig. 4.21). This may be considered an additional aid to lubrication and is referred to as an *elastohydrodynamic* phenomenon. It was initially described when rubber coatings were put on steel rollers. Elastohydrodynamic effects help lower the coefficient of friction in articular joints and the elasticity of the bearing surface helps the surface bunch up at the edges to keep the fluid within the zone of impending contact.

---

*The squeezing together of the two bearing surfaces creates pressurization of any fluid lubricant caught between the surfaces. The resulting fluid film of lubricant is called a squeeze film.

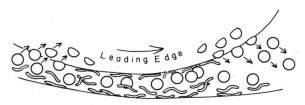

Figure 4.20. In joints under load the fluid film between the cartilage surfaces is composed of wept interstitial fluid and trapped synovial fluid. Under most physiologic circumstances the fluid weeps out at the leading edge of contact. Osmotic pressure pulls the interstitial fluid back into the cartilage substance in unloaded areas, usually at the trailing edge.

During a normal cycle of joint motion one would expect the prevalent lubricating mechanism to change from predominantly boundary to predominantly "weeping" back to predominantly boundary with a combination of both mechanisms active during most of the load and motion cycle.

The effectiveness of this range of lubricating mechanisms over the range of loads and motion encountered in normal joints is demonstrated in Fig. 4.22, which compares the friction, which is a direct indicator of lubricating effectiveness, of the synovial joint under different loads. From the figure note that synovial tissue rubbing over articular cartilage or synovial tissue rubbing on itself has a frictional resistance considerably higher than that encountered in cartilage on cartilage lubrication. This is because synovial tissue does not permit the full range of lubricating mechanisms that occur when cartilage is lubricated with synovial fluid. Not enough pressure is exerted to allow for a hydrostatic phenomenon and the relatively slow velocity of sliding as well as its oscillatory nature precludes a hydrodynamic phenomenon. Synovial tissue rubbing on itself is primarily lubricated by synovial fluid hyaluronate which adheres to the synovial tissue and provides a boundary type of lubrication.

The presence of this large molecule, hyaluronate, whose major function is the boundary lubrication of soft tissue, gives synovial fluid significant viscous resistance to flow. The shear forces created by these large, ungainly molecules is significant in that they entangle and entrap each other as the fluid flows (Fig. 4.23). It takes a certain amount of shear to move these molecules along and this gives the fluid its viscous properties. This entrapment of molecules is obviously less if the fluid flows quickly and is what is meant by *thixotropy*.

Ketchup is a common thixotropic fluid. One pounds on the ketchup bottle to

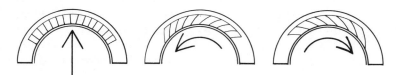

Figure 4.21. The elasticity of the surfaces can aid in lowering the functional resistance. This is referred to as an elastohydrodynamic effect.

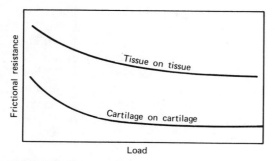

Figure 4.22. Friction as a function of load for cartilage on cartilage, and synovial tissue on synovial tissue.

increase the velocity of the flow. Although a thixotropic lubricant, particularly at low shear rates, adds to the frictional resistance of joints, this incremental increase is well worth accepting because the viscous nature of the lubricant provides it with significant spreading powers. This is particularly the case when one is concerned with lubrication of soft tissue, which because of its many folds and convolutions might otherwise frequently be without a fluid film or means of obtaining a lubricant during a particular attitude or function of a joint if the synovial fluid flowed about too freely. The viscous nature of the synovial fluid maintains it spread around in all recesses of the synovium.

7. ATTEMPTS TO TREAT OSTEOARTHROSIS WITH ARTIFICIAL LUBRICANTS

An understanding of the normal lubricating mechanisms shows that joint lubrication depends on the presence of cartilage for both the hydrostatic and boundary lubricating mechanisms to function. Particularly under high loads the hyd-

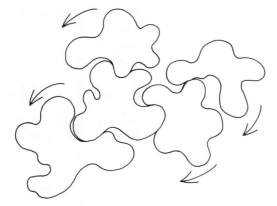

Figure 4.23. The viscous nature of synovial fluid is the result of the entanglement of hyaluronate molecules.

rostatic (weeping) mechanism is the crucial friction-lowering device. These facts suggest that artificial lubricants, in the presence of mildly destroyed cartilage, are of little use. The addition of oil or silicone blocks the free flow of water in and out of cartilage, effectively destroying the important hydrostatic mechanism.

Attempts to add appropriate boundary lubricating molecules have so far been thwarted by an inability to produce molecules that are both hydrophilic and not immediately cleared from the synovial space. The concept that what arthritic joints need is a "good grease job" misrepresents the true situation. The osteoarthrotic joint needs a functioning articular surface.

GLOSSARY

Boundary lubrication   Separation of bearing surfaces by a film of lubricant that adheres to the surfaces themselves. Also dry friction where asperities of high points of the two bearing surfaces touch when rubbed. This latter definition is in a strict engineering sense and does not apply to a joint that always contains a film of fluid lubricant.

Coefficient of friction   A parameter used to relate frictional resistance of two objects rubbing on each other, determined by dividing the frictional force by the compressive load across the bearing.

Elasticity   Deformation of an object when the stress depends only on the magnitude of the strain, independent of the rate at which the object is being strained or deformed. When the stress is removed, the strain disappears.

Elastohydrodynamic lubrication   Relates the various frictional lowering advantages obtained when the bearing surfaces are elastic in nature.

Hydrodynamic lubrication   Situation where the two bearing surfaces are separated by a fluid film held in place by the relative motion of the two bearing surfaces.

Hydrostatic lubrication   Creation of a fluid film by pressurizing the fluid.

Partial body mass   Mass part of the body, for example the mass acting on the hip joint on the swing side in gait, is a partial body mass as the weight of the swing leg distal to that hip is not being supported by that hip.

Thixotropy   Viscosity that is shear rate dependent.

Viscoelasticity   When stress depends on the rate of strain as well as the magnitude of the strain.

Weeping lubrication   Special form of hydrostatic lubrication (see above) in which the interstitial fluid of cartilage is pressed out into the joint space by the deformation of cartilage under load.

5
Joint Replacements

1. GENERAL REMARKS

The concept that "worn out" joints can be replaced by mechanical bearings is an attractive one and some clinical success has been achieved. In general, replacement of a destroyed joint with an artificial one significantly changes the nature and distribution of stress within the system. Several serious mechanical problems can result from these changes, which can lead to failure of the materials that have been implanted or an extreme biological response.

As described in Chapter 4, the normal joint functions with an extremely low frictional resistance and maintains a maximal contact area under almost all circumstances because the articulating bearing surfaces and their underlying bone can deform. Shear created at the interfaces between cartilage and bone is minimized and the position of the joint components is optimal.

The lubrication mechanisms of plastic-on-metal bearing surfaces are not similar to those of the normal joint; the frictional resistance of total joint replacements is higher. Total joint replacements are generally subjected to the same external forces due to body weight, muscle force, and impulsive loads from the activities of daily living which apply to natural joints. The conformation of natural joints depends upon the compliance of articular cartilage and underlying subchondral bone. Such compliance is absent in a total joint replacement. The shock-absorbing features provided by the cancellous bone and metaphyseal cortical bone in normal joints are absent when the joint is replaced by relatively much stiffer plastic, metal, or bone-cement composites. These relatively inelastic materials, compared to living tissues, create significant problems and have a profound effect on the service life of total joint replacement.

It is necessary to anchor the prosthesis to the skeleton. If the prosthesis were completely free to move it might dislocate, subluxate, or have limited contact with bone. Limited contact creates local concentrations of stress which erode the underlying bone. Fixation of the joint replacement to the skeleton has been most successful with polymethyl methacrylate, so-called "bone cement," grouting material that "cements" the prosthesis not by adhesion (it is not adhesive) but by interdigitation with adjoining bone. This interdigitation, if complete, fixes the prosthesis (Fig. 5.1).

The eventual generation of a fibrous layer in the interface, and various degrees of loosening create significant changes in the stress distribution on the prosthetic replacement and the bone into which it is attached. The mechanical success of total joint replacement depends on the specific mechanical situation

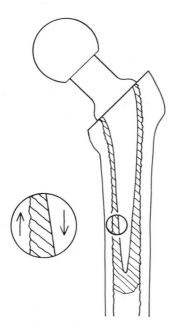

Figure 5.1. Shear stresses are transmitted from the prosthesis shank to the endosteum.

that one is trying to substitute for. To explain this we have elected to discuss primarily hip and knee joint replacements, first by presenting design specifications for replacement and then evaluating current models. The success of approximating these mechanical requirements is vastly different for these two different joints. The point of this chapter, utilizing primarily these two examples, is to demonstrate that the success of total joint replacement depends on completely understanding the biomechanical requirements of the joint being replaced and the effects prosthetic replacement has on the remaining skeleton.

2.   STRESSES IN THE NORMAL HIP JOINT

In normal joints the pattern of stress distribution depends upon the magnitude and position of the overall force transmitted through the joint. The coefficient of friction of normal joints is so low that forces parallel to the surface (shear forces) are negligible.

The loading pattern on the femoral head and acetabulum is primarily composed of compressive forces and subjects the subchondral bone near the joint to a compressive stress distribution. In the acetabulum, compressive stresses at the surface of the joint decrease as they radiate out from the concave surface of the acetabulum, because they must be borne by greater and greater areas of bone within the pelvis (Fig. 5.2).

In the femoral head the opposite is true (Fig. 5.3). The stresses increase as the compressive force radiates in from the convex surface of the femoral head. The neck and shaft of the femur have considerably smaller cross-sectional areas than does the femoral head and the stresses are transmitted down to the femoral shaft

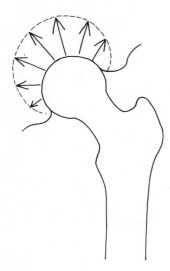

Figure 5.2. In the normal hip joint, stresses transmitted from the femoral head to the acetabulum radiate out and decrease in magnitude as they are transmitted into the pelvis.

through the femoral neck passing into smaller areas of bone, resulting in stresses of higher magnitude within the neck than in the femoral head.

The stress distribution and types of stresses in the femoral neck and shaft are also altered by the fact that the resultant force acting on the femoral head is not parallel to the axis of the neck (Fig. 5.4). The bending moment so created establishes a stress distribution of compressive stresses in the medial inferior aspect of the neck and tensile stresses in the lateral superior aspect of the neck (Fig. 5.5). These stresses increase in magnitude as they progress from the joint toward the base of the femoral neck, as the bending moment is increased. Note that the entire neck is still subjected to some compressive stress since a component of the resultant force is still directed along the axis of the neck (Fig. 5.6).

This compressive stress adds to the compressive stress as a result of the bending stresses in the medial inferior aspect of the neck and decreases the tensile stresses in the lateral superior aspect of the neck (Fig. 5.7).

The stresses due to bending are greater in magnitude than are the stresses from pure compression. If the femoral neck is directed in a line more parallel to the resultant compressive force, in other words more in valgus, the bending

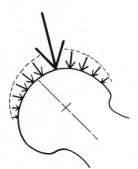

Figure 5.3. The stress distribution resulting from the total resultant force on the normal femoral head is compressive and well distributed over the femoral head.

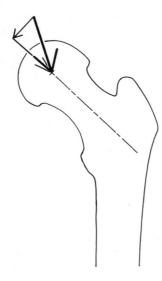

Figure 5.4. The resultant force on the femoral head has components along and perpendicular to the femoral neck axis.

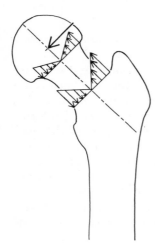

Figure 5.5. Bending stress distribution in the femoral neck due to the perpendicular components of the joint force. Note compression medially and tension laterally.

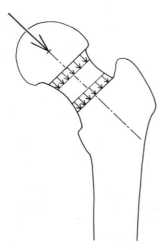

Figure 5.6. The stress in the femoral neck due to the axial component is compressive.

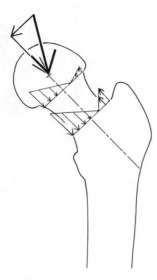

Figure 5.7. The combination of bending and compressive stress in the femoral neck acts to decrease the tensile stress in the lateral aspect of the neck .

moment within the neck would be decreased or even eliminated. In such a situation only the relatively small stresses from compression would remain. Keep in mind that such alterations in types of stresses and stress patterns can occur with the same overall resultant joint force.

The abductor muscle creates a force that acts generally upward at the intertrochanteric level. Because the femoral neck sits eccentrically, the abductors produce their own bending moment. Their effect is to increase the tensile stresses laterally and the compressive stresses medially (Fig. 5.8). At every level of the femoral shaft, the overall force on the bone results from the force exerted by the partial body mass and from the muscles acting at this level. It has been shown that the femur is stressed in bending in a plane close to the frontal plane (Fig. 5.9). The bending stress decreases from the hip toward the knee where it is replaced by pure compressive stress.

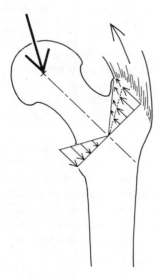

Figure 5.8. The force created by the abductors tends to increase both the compressive and tensile stresses in the femoral neck.

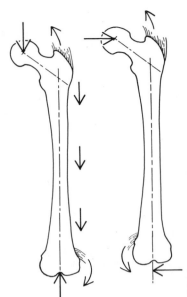

Figure 5.9. The hip joint and abductor forces tend to bend the femoral shaft.

3.   STRESS DISTRIBUTION AFTER TOTAL HIP REPLACEMENT

Let us consider the stress distribution pattern after total joint replacement. First, remember that the shear forces developed at the joint surface are no longer negligible and produce torques which can act to loosen the prosthesis where it is attached to the bone. Secondly, the size and position of the contact areas between prosthesis and bone are crucial in determining the type and magnitude of the stresses developed. Third, the materials that compose the replacement have different moduli of elasticity consequently altering the relationship between the stresses and strains developed.

If we consider prosthetic replacement at the hip joint with total contact between the femoral and acetabular components, the normal forces developed at the joint surface again produce a similar pattern of compressive forces radiating out into the prosthetic acetabulum and concentrating within the femoral head. Being less compliant than bone, the acetabular component has less of a tendency to distribute the stress it is transmitting. In comparison to a normal bony acetabulum, greater than the normal compressive stresses arise in the superior area of the cup and less than normal compressive stresses arise in its medial aspect (Fig. 5.10).

If the femoral component contacts the acetabular component centrally, the latter is not significantly subjected to bending. However, with hip motion the resultant joint force tends to act more toward the periphery of the acetabular component, tending to bend it (Fig. 5.11). The resulting strains in the acetabular component can promote loosening. If the forces are transmitted through a small central contact area (femoral head diameter less than acetabular diameter), since the force is the same and the area is decreased, the surface compressive stresses

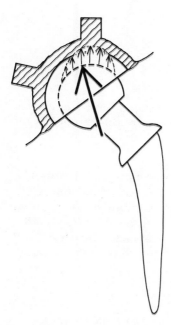

Figure 5.10. The general stress distribution in the acetabular component due to joint force is mainly compressive.

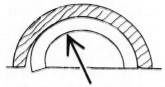 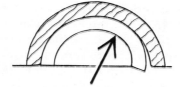

Figure 5.11. Under an oscillating joint force the acetabular component has a tendency to be bent (exaggerated in this figure).

noted above are increased (Fig. 5.12). The pattern of stress in the cup is similar to that with total contact but is now more exaggerated. If the forces are transmitted through a horseshoe-shaped circular contact area located about the periphery of the ball, as shown in Fig. 5.13, the local stresses developed in the area of the contacting surface are again increased but the tendency to central apical bending of the acetabular component is reduced, or may even be reversed (Fig. 5.13).

Regardless of whether one considers the local contact stresses at the surface or

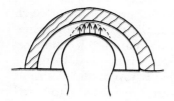

Figure 5.12. Stresses increase when the femoral head is smaller than the acetabular component.

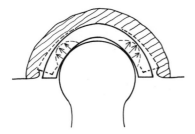

Figure 5.13. When the femoral head size exceeds that of the cup the stresses are concentrated at the periphery of the cup.

the overall stresses within the cup, the effect on the prosthetic material cannot be considered merely as static and unchanging. Since joint forces are intermittent in magnitude and the resulting vector with joint motion continually shifts in its location, the magnitude and pattern of the stresses and strains developed in the material are also continually changing. Thus an additional fact to be considered in the design of any prosthesis is the fatigue life of the implanted material, cement, and bone.

4.   PROSTHETIC ACETABULAR STRESS DISTRIBUTION AND JOINT SHEAR FORCE

In addition to compressive joint forces the acetabulum also is subject to and transmits shear forces created at the joint surface. Unlike the normal cartilage-surfaced articulation, which has almost no frictional resistance, the prosthetic "low friction" prosthesis has a coefficient of friction that can be 40 to 50 times greater than that of the normal joint. This frictional resistance creates modest shear forces at the interface. Although these shear forces are much lower than the existing compressive forces, they must be included in any consideration of the mechanical effects in joint replacements. The role of shear forces on the acetabular component affects the contact stresses of the material in the vicinity of the joint and the stress distribution pattern throughout the material.

The shear forces alter the angle of the resultant stresses generated toward the direction of movement since near the surface of the joint the shear forces are perpendicular to the compressive forces (Fig. 5.14). The material being compressed in one direction must therefore deform; tensile stresses and strains result (Fig. 5.15). This effect decreases the further away from the surface one examines the stresses. If the shear forces are of a sufficient magnitude, the material being compressed in the direction of movement could tend to shift in this direction.

Over a period of time if one examines the surface of a used polyethylene acetabular component one may note that the surface material is deformed. This deformation occurs slowly and may be described as "creep" or "cold flow." Such a phenomenon can happen only if the material is sufficiently plastic or deformable. It thins out where the compressive forces are maximal and accumulates where the compressive stresses are minimal. If the material is not as deformable or if the rate at which the forces are applied is sufficiently rapid, tensile strains break the material apart rather than cause it to simply deform, as has happened with some polyester and ceramic acetabular components.

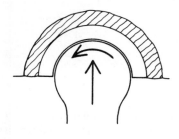

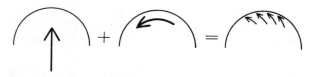

Figure 5.14. The frictional (shear) forces are, at the surface, perpendicular to the compressive forces. The shear forces tend to alter the angle of the resultant stresses toward the direction in which the joint is moving.

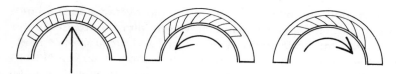

Figure 5.15. Materials being compressed in one direction must deform. Tensile stresses and strains result. The reversal of motion sets the stage for creep or tensile fatigue of the acetabular component. (Note that this is the same as Figure 4.21 but with a very different caption, pointing up the dramatic differences between the mechanical behavior of polyethylene and articular cartilage.)

5. STRESSES IN THE ACETABULAR CEMENT–SUBCHONDRAL BONE INTERFACE

The effects of the stress distribution pattern in the acetabular component of a joint replacement are threefold:

- Possible mechanical failure of the acetabulum. To date, strains developed in the presently used acetabular components do not appear to be a common clinical problem.
- Prosthetic replacements do not absorb energy as well as a normal joint. With total joint replacement more energy is transmitted to the peripheral bony bed.
- Perhaps most important is alteration in the forces transmitted to the peripheral cement-bone interface.

The stresses generated at the cement-bone interface surrounding the acetabular component are obviously the result of the compressive and shear forces at the hip joint surface altered by their transmission through the acetabular component. In general, because the joint forces are directed predominantly superior

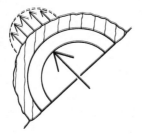

Figure 5.16. The superior and medial aspect of the bone-cement interface is primarily subject to compressive stress.

and medial, this area of cement and bone primarily is subject to compressive stresses (Fig. 5.16). However, since the medial and lateral aspects of this interface are more parallel to the direction of major (compressive) force transmission, these areas are subject to shear forces (Fig. 5.17).

The greater the concentration of forces in a superior direction, the greater the shear forces on the medial and lateral sides. Such shear forces can almost be as high in magnitude as the resultant joint force itself. Since the compressive forces are intermittent, the shear stresses they produce oscillate. As long as the prosthetic surfaces retain low frictional resistance they contribute only slightly to the cement-bone interface shear.

In general, the direction and magnitude of forces on the subchondral bone are similar to those in the cement. Two factors, however, alter the stresses in the bone. First is the relationship between the type of force and the area of cement-contact through which it is transmitted. In areas where there is no cement between the bone and the acetabular component, shear forces developed are not transmitted to the bone. In addition, even in areas where cement exists, there may not be good contact between the two, since cement is not an adhesive, and depends upon interdigitations with the bone to transmit shear stress. Thus at the bone-cement interface although the area over which compressive forces are distributed in the subchondral bone is equal to or greater than that in the cement, the area over which the shear forces are distributed can be less. Thus, considerable stress concentrations can arise at this interface.

The second factor that enters into the development of the stresses created at the subchondral bone-cement interface is the architecture of the subchondral bone itself. As cancellous bone is porous, the total area of bone involved is less than the outer circumferential area of the acetabular cup-cement interface. Thus the magnitude of the stresses evoked in any trabeculum is probably greater than that in the adjacent cement. Further, since each trabeculum of bone now is not necessarily aligned in an optimal orientation to resist the new stress distribution

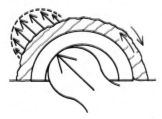

Figure 5.17. The medial and lateral aspects of the bone-cement interface are subject to shear, even if the femoral head is not in contact in these areas.

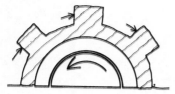

Figure 5.18. Adding "pegs" of cement to the acetabular fixation increases its resistance to shear.

pattern, the type of stress is highly dependent on the trabecular orientation relative to the transmitted force.

It is therefore easy to understand why mechanical failure on the acetabular side of a total hip replacement usually occurs at the bone-cement interface. The surgeon may limit the magnitude of the stress in the acetabular bone-cement interface by: (1) insuring a cement interface which has contact with trabecular material, rather than the inner cortical table of the pelvis, (2) putting as much cement as possible about the entire acetabulum in direct contact with as many trabeculae as possible, and (3) drilling holes into the acetabulum filled with cement (Fig. 5.18). All these measures increase the area of bone receiving the forces; hence, the stresses are reduced.

6. STRESS DISTRIBUTION IN THE FEMORAL PROSTHESIS

The compressive forces developed at the femoral prosthetic joint surface produce compressive stresses in the prosthesis as in a normal femoral head although the stress and distribution may be altered. The factors cited in our discussion of the acetabular side affecting the stress pattern—contacting area, location of contact, geometry, and type of material employed—play a role in dictating the overall stress distribution.

When considering just the stresses locally present at the surface, the same factors of force magnitude and total contact area affect the stresses here as they do on the acetabular side. In the neck and shank of the femoral prosthesis, the compressive force eccentrically located at the base of the spherical head creates a pattern of predominantly compressive and bending stresses similar to those noted in the normal femoral neck and trochanteric regions.

Any changes in geometry of the femoral prosthesis itself that alter the neck length (ie, the eccentricity of the compressive loading forces in relation to the axis of the neck), modify the bending stresses in the shank. Reducing the neck length or designing a more valgus oriented prosthesis creates a more uniform compressive stress pattern in the shank because it decreases the bending stress (Fig. 5.19). This effectively decreases the compressive stresses on the medial side of the shank and the tensile stresses on the lateral side. The magnitude of the stresses within the shank also depends on the cross-sectional area of the shank and the distribution of the material present considered in reference to its neutral axis, that is, the area moment of inertia of the material in the shank, particularly on the medial (compressive) side. The greater the amount of cross-sectional material, the lower the stress per unit volume as the total force is distributed over

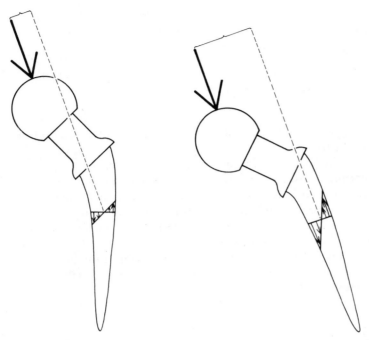

Figure 5.19. Increasing the valgus of the prosthetic femoral neck (*left*) decreases the bending stress in the shank.

a greater area. The greater the cross-sectional area medial to the neutral axis, the lower the compressive stress and the higher the tensile stress (Fig. 5.20).

A sharply angulated shank can act as a stress concentrator which under intermittent loading can fatigue the prosthesis as high stresses are created on both the tensile and compressive sides. Ultimately the strains that develop in the material and its resistance to failure are dependent on these factors plus the material properties (modulus of elasticity, ultimate tensile stress, and fatigue strength) of the component itself.

7.   STRESSES IN THE FEMORAL PROSTHESIS SECONDARY TO FIXATION

The femoral component is subjected to stresses from both compression and bending. The bending stresses in the prosthesis are the most potentially disastrous. Bending creates tensile stresses laterally, which, since loading is intermittent, can initiate and propagate cracks and stem fracture. The manner and degree to which the femoral component is constrained drastically alter the pattern and magnitude of the stresses developed in and about its neck and shaft. If bone or cement fixes the prosthesis about its shank alone, leaving the prosthetic collar unsupported (Fig. 5.21), the bending moment and stress created within the prosthesis are greater than if contact is made between the prosthesis and calcar. Failure could occur either in the prosthetic stem or in the surrounding cement, which is subjected to considerable stress.

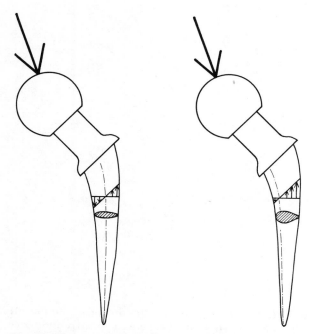

Figure 5.20. The amount and distribution of the cross-sectional area of the femoral component shank play a significant role in the stress distribution in the stem.

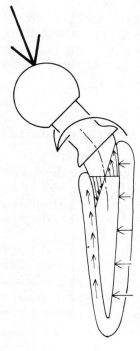

Figure 5.21. When the prosthetic collar is unsupported, increased bending stresses are created within the femoral stem. The surrounding cement is also under significant stress.

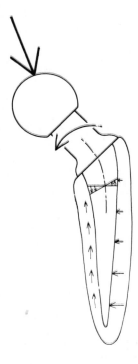

Figure 5.22. Supporting the prosthetic collar significantly lowers the bending stress in the stem. The surrounding cement is under less stress than in the situation in Fig. 5.21.

If the prosthesis is bearing load on the calcar, although the compressive stresses in the region of the calcar are increased, the bending stresses in the shank are decreased as the moment arm is decreased (Fig. 5.22).

If the compressive stresses transmitted from the femoral head are concentrated in the stem because of poor fixation of the prosthesis along its shank, there is no opposing force from surrounding cement or bone except at the shank *tip*. What happens in such a case is a stress concentration in the shank, with resultant failure from tensile fatigue (Fig. 5.23).

8. FORCES AND STRESSES IN THE CEMENT AND BONE SURROUNDING THE FEMORAL PROSTHESIS

The stresses created in the cement and bone on the femoral side are highly dependent upon the shape, size, and position of the prosthesis, as well as the location, orientation, and amount of contact between it and the surrounding cement and bone. Though joint shear forces contribute somewhat, the compressive forces contribute the most to the bending moment created.

The advantage of a low friction over a higher friction design is that less muscular force is required to move the apposing surfaces relative to one another. This lessens the force on the joint in both shear and compression. Regardless of how the bending moment is created, if loosening of the prosthesis is to be prevented, the bending moment must be resisted by forces generated mainly by

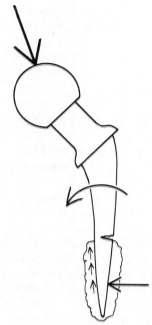

Figure 5.23. Inadequate fixation of the femoral component in its proximal portions can lead to fatigue failure of the prosthetic stem.

the bone-cement interface proximal-medially and distal-laterally. Compressive forces generated in these areas can be transmitted across this interface, but proximal-lateral and distal-medial tensile forces cannot be transmitted; only separation of the surfaces in these areas occurs. If settling is to be prevented, the compressive joint force having a component directed down the prosthesis must be resisted by forces generated at the collar and prosthetic tip, as well as along the prosthetic shank.

Attempts to reduce the bending moment by decreasing the degree of varus in the prosthesis or decreasing the neck length chosen, increase the compressive component of the forces transmitted down the prosthetic shaft. This consequently increases the compressive stresses generated in the area of cement and bone about the collar and prosthetic tip, as well as increasing the shear forces along the shank.

Marked decreases in stresses, on the other hand, could well lead to osteoporosis with secondary early degradation of the bone-cement interface and an increased incidence of loosening. Thus, more massive femoral components may cause different problems, such as an area of stress concentration at the junction between the distal end of this section and the remainder of the femur. In such a case, a single incident of high force secondary to trauma would not be needed to cause failure, as a fatigue fracture through the junction of the stiffened and nonstiffened sections could occur, much as the spine is subjected to spondylolysis just above or below a spinal fusion (see Chapter 1). We do not know how much the increased stiffness of such new prostheses affects the service life of the cement-bone interface or prosthetic-bone femoral-shaft junction.

Thus, although the cross-sectional area of a femoral stem must be large enough to withstand bending stresses which it is subjected to, too large a stem may not be in the patient's best interest.

Regardless of the inherent shape of the prosthesis, the surgeon still provides for its final position within the shaft and the degree to which it is surrounded by cement and bone. Thus to a great extent, successful fixation of the femoral components depends upon the surgical technique of insertion. Ideally, a complete bone-cement interface surrounds the collar and shank to distribute whatever forces are present over as wide an area as possible. If there is no contact between the femoral components' collar and calcar by direct apposition or by the interposition of cement, the shear and bending forces transmitted to the area below this level are increased (Fig. 5.24).

These increased bending forces plus the compressive forces now not resisted by a collar must be resisted by the materials about the shaft and tip. The bending moment is the most potentially damaging to the cement surrounding the prosthesis stem. Compressive stresses in the cement increase proximal-medially and distal-laterally. Adjacent bone is subjected to stresses in a transverse direction (primarily medial-lateral). The structure of cortical bone in this area is not oriented in a direction that offers a significant resistance to stress in this direction. It can provide for this only after remodeling occurs, a process that, if it occurs, would take a long time. More likely, in the interim the absence of longitudinal stress could cause osteopenia and produce a weak bony structure.

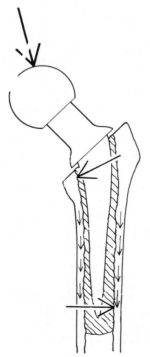

Figure 5.24. If there is no contact between the collar and calcar, stresses at the cement-bone interface increase proximal-medially and distal-laterally due to the bending moment.

Compressive stresses are then concentrated within the cement and trabecular bone surrounding the prosthetic stem.

The high concentration of stresses produced is further aggravated by the fact that this same region in the absence of calcar contact must also resist the compressive forces transmitted down the prosthesis. Because the interface area is parallel to these forces, they are transmitted to the cement and adjacent trabecular bone as shear stresses. As the orientation of the trabecular bone is not maximally oriented to receive stresses in this direction, it is unclear how much of this stress the interface can stand, and failure can occur.

If reaming removes the trabecular bone, only cement offers resistance to the joint forces generated. It is thus obviously beneficial to the surgeon to retain as much endosteal trabecular bone as possible. The cement must also be sufficient in volume to extend to and below the end of the prosthesis to ensure as large an area as possible over which the forces can be distributed. Any decrease in the cement-bone surface contact area increases the stresses in the remaining area of contact. Any movement of the prosthesis during cement hardening is to be avoided, since the forces are transmitted from the prosthesis to the cement only in the area of high spots where contact occurs. Sufficient cement must be used to ensure as wide and complete an infiltration of the grouting material into the endosteal trabecular bone as possible. This is especially important in maintaining the cement-bone interface's resistance to shear forces created. Without sufficient interdigitation, little of the shear forces is resisted by the trabecular bone along the shaft, and the cement toward and below the tip of the stem is forced to resist all the joint forces tending to sink the prosthesis.

On the other hand, attempts to overpressurize the cement can cause infusion pressure or temperature sufficient to cause osteonecrosis of the endosteal trabecular bone, eventually leading to resorption. Replacement of this bone by fibrous tissue creates a situation similar to having reamed out the trabecular bone, which for all practical purposes offers no resistance to movement and prosthetic loosening.

Providing contact between the prosthetic collar and calcar (Fig. 5.25), or interposing a layer of cement in this area (Fig. 5.26), greatly helps to reduce the stresses borne by the cement and trabecular bone along the shaft. Both the bending moments, as well as the compressive load transmitted down the shaft, are reduced. The overall joint force is now shared by a greater area. Furthermore, in almost all areas the stresses generated in the bone-cement complex are primarily compressive and are maximal medially, the type and location which can best be resisted by such materials. Ideally, a complete bone-cement interface surrounding the shank should still remain to distribute these compressive stresses as widely as possible. In its absence, the brunt of the stresses is borne in the region of the calcar.

At the time of this writing, fragmentation of the cement, when it is interposed between the prosthetic collar and the calcar, and resorption of the calcar in the absence of cement have both been clinically noted. It is easy to see how such circumstances imply high stress concentrations and possible subsequent fatigue failure. Resorption of the calcar is a telltale sign of loosening or prosthetic settling.

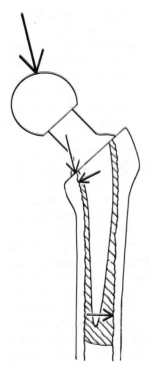

Figure 5.25. Providing contact between the collar and the calcar reduces the stresses in the cement and bone.

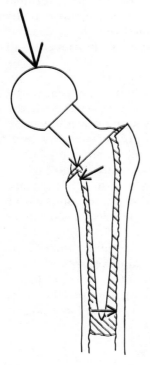

Figure 5.26. Stresses are reduced by interposing a layer of cement between the prosthetic collar and the calcar.

9. KNEE JOINT STABILITY—NEWTON REVISITED

The stability of a joint is dependent upon the fact that forces acting in given directions are prevented from causing motion or are allowed to create motion but under controlled conditions of speed and distance. Three mechanisms at each joint maintain stability: cartilage and bony geometry, muscular action, and ligamentous resistance. The degree to which each mechanism contributes varies with the joint in question.

In the knee the factors that determine the stability are somewhat different from those at the hip. The ball and socket geometry of the hip prevents any translational motion but fully permits rotation in any arc about a central fixed axis. Dynamic stability is needed only to control this motion, not to limit any direction except extension. Thus, except anteriorly, ligaments in the hip joint play a small role, and muscle tension in almost all planes is required to balance the acetabular cup on the femoral head. Total hip relplacement does little to alter these normal mechanisms of stability.

The knee is a flexural linkage with mandatory associated rotations that must bear as much load and be as stable as the hip. But the demands of motion are different and the three parameters stabilizing the joint contribute differently than those at the hip. Flexion-extension, abduction-adduction, and internal-external rotation occur simultaneously around three axes of rotation which are not fixed. Motion may be translational as well as rotational.

To provide for such freedom of motion, so restrictive a bony contour as that at the hip is not permissible at the knee. To allow some motion in certain directions but limit the range, ligaments play a larger role here than at the hip. To control the speed of such motions, especially when high torques are present (bending, jumping, going up and down stairs), muscles are not only needed, but require the assistance of changing lever arms to maximize the counteracting torques they can develop. Thus, stability is achieved by a combination of surface contours, collateral and cruciate ligaments, and posterior joint capsule, that act together to permit, yet limit, motion and provide optimal lever arms for the activated muscles.

The relative importance of each factor varies with the motion specified. For example, in the frontal plane, medial-lateral translational motion is restricted by the projecting tibial spines (Fig. 5.27). The force due to the body mass creating

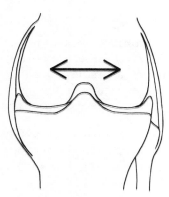

Figure 5.27. Medial-lateral translation of the knee is limited by the tibial spines.

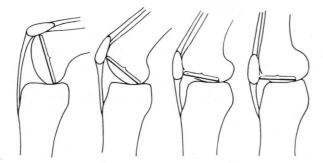

Figure 5.28. The lever arms of the muscles about the knee change with knee position. Note the decrease in lever arm of the quadriceps with extension, as the torque required from that muscle is decreased.

varus torque is limited in creating movement primarily by the lateral collateral ligaments and lateral muscular stay. In the sagittal plane, the demands of controlling high body torques during large flexion-extension excursions requires large muscle masses and continually changing lever arms provided by the nonspherical (multiaxis) femoral condyles (Fig. 5.28).

To provide for this, anterior-posterior translational motion cannot be restricted by tibial contouring; some sliding motion thereby accompanies the rotation and is limited by strong cruciate ligaments, collateral ligaments, and at certain points the posterior capsule.

Deterioration of the knee joint has a dual effect; it causes a change in the bony contours of the joint surface and alters ligament lengths. Surgical replacement of the bony contours of the knee is thus more difficult than that at the hip, since substitution must be made for the lack of stability due to bony as well as ligamentous deterioration. Although several hundred designs for knee replacements have been fabricated, all fall into three main categories: unconstrained, constrained, and semi-constrained. We shall examine the mechanical ramifications of these designs.

10. JOINT CONTACT STRESSES IN UNCONSTRAINED KNEE PROSTHESES

Effect of Design

In many patients whose knee would seem suitable for prosthetic replacement, the ligaments are still intact. One should theoretically have to insert only two nonconnected components to achieve stability. Under such a circumstance the degree of stability actually achieved is dependent on (1) tightness of the ligaments when inserting the prosthetic components and (2) the surface contour of the prosthetic elements themselves.

The common materials in use are, as in hip replacements, noncorrosive metal on polyethylene. Polyethylene, even the ultra-high molecular weight version used in such applications, as any plastic, deforms under relatively low stress.

Therefore the surface interface between the metal and plastic must be maximal to avoid exceeding the elastic limit of the polyethylene and causing it to creep or cold flow and deform.

In the hip, maximal contact areas occur at all attitudes of the joint within its range of motions. The knee slides as well as glides: therefore, total or maximal contact may not always occur. A design with femoral and tibial components of exactly the same radius provides maximal contact area within the limited range of flexion such a design provides, but does not allow for axial rotation or abduction/adduction. In such a case all sideways motion and rotation would be restrained by the tibial component's prosthetic walls. Forces developed in abduction/adduction and in rotation would be high in this region, especially if the grooved wall did not have as large a contact area as possible. In most cases the walls on the tibial side are made of polyethylene and have a lower yield strength than metal femoral components. Besides cold flow (Fig. 5.29), fractures can occur in the polyethylene area from either single force insults which exceed the ultimate strength of the material or by repeated less-than-ultimate yield forces which can create failure by fatigue.

Making the tibial components flat, like a sled, allows more freedom of motion and allows the knee to slide, but doing so creates stress concentrations (Fig. 5.30) and transfers the entire role of stabilizing the joint onto the ligaments, which are susceptible to stretching out with a subsequent loss of stability, more sliding, and eventual subluxation or dislocation.

The demand put on the designer of knee prostheses with regard to surface contour alone is more critical and more difficult than for hip prostheses. A finer balance must exist between concessions made to surface geometry and ligaments in tension in order to prevent failure of ligament stability or of prosthesis material due to either high stresses because of small contact areas or motion restrictions due to alterations in overall contour.

Not only is it difficult to design the maximum shape and contact area but also it is difficult for the surgeon to assess the functional length of the ligaments and to insert the right size prosthesis to maintain these ligaments in a position to share the load with the prosthesis.

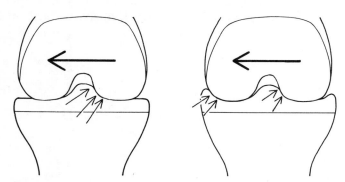

Figure 5.29. Attempts to constrain knee motion with tibial shapes of polyethylene lead to cold flow of the material (and sometimes fracture) due to the stress concentrations.

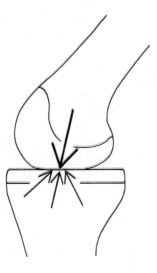

Figure 5.30. Sled-like shapes for tibial components lead to stress concentrations in the polyethylene.

Effects of Alignment

Since these prostheses are not constrained, the surgeon can alter the alignment in a variety of ways which markedly change the magnitude and type of forces as well as their distribution across the knee joint. Uncorrected varus angulation or laxity in the lateral ligaments increases the compressive forces on the medial side (Fig. 5.31). Bending moments create increased compressive stresses in the material on the medial side and increased tension in the ligaments on the lateral side. This may reduce or neutralize the overall compressive force of the normal joint force on the lateral side, or if it is large enough, actually create tension in the lateral ligaments.

Valgus angulation, on the other hand, can produce significant alterations by completely altering the bending moment so as to cause high compressive forces on the lateral side and tension on the medial ligament.

Ligament length as well as strength may be so altered because of the disease as to not permit full correction. For example, in rheumatoid arthritis the medial collateral ligament can be quite good compared to the lateral which may be short

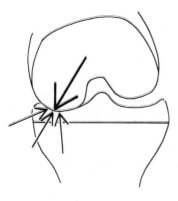

Figure 5.31. Laxity leading to angulation of knee replacements creates stress concentrations.

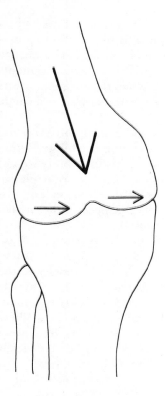

Figure 5.32. If valgus angulation occurs with an inclination of the joint line, shear forces result as the joint tries to sublux.

and weak. One may want to maintain some of this rather than overcorrect into varus or one may not be able to totally correct the malalignment.

The delicate balance between these factors of angulation versus ligament tautness and strength varies from case to case. Forces across the joint so altered in magnitude and distribution may not necessarily yield compressive or tensile stresses but may create greater shear forces and stresses depending on the over-all angulation of the joint surface itself relative to a vertical line (Fig. 5.32). In such a case stresses are dependent on the total contact area and the degree of inclination of the joint surface.

An additional factor is introduced as the stresses depend on whether or not these two areas come in contact with their opposing surfaces at the same time. If they do not, the one that comes in contact first bears the total amount of stress and the other one bears none. This condition may or may not exist, depending on whether the design has separate medial and lateral compartment components or two connected components. If the former is the case, the importance of the surgeon's placement cannot be overemphasized.

11.   STRESSES IN CONSTRAINED PROSTHESES

The need for an inherently stable prosthetic knee, which maintains stability in the absence of cruciate and/or collateral ligaments, is apparent. A number of totally constrained hinge prostheses have been developed to meet this need.

The most constrained knee joint prosthesis has a hinge that allows only a single motion: flexion/extension (Fig. 5.33). Because of this hinge, the relationship of the femoral component to the tibial component is constant. The degree of varus/valgus angulation and anterior/posterior position of the components with regard to each other is fixed by the manufacturer. When the surgeon inserts the prosthesis, he can alter only the alignment of the entire prosthesis as a single unit.

The large anterior-posterior shear forces related to load-bearing on a moving knee replaced with a hinge prosthesis are transmitted through the hinge. These are added to the normal joint forces which are at least 3 to 4 times body weight and are accentuated in gait by the bending moment created by the relative medial placement of the body's center of gravity vis-à-vis the knee. For this reason the maximum compressive stress is on the superior aspect on the medial side and the inferior aspect on the lateral side of the hinge (Fig. 5.34).

The compressive forces are transmitted between the femoral component on the midportion of the bolt's superior surface while the compressive forces transmitted between the tibial component and the bolt are transmitted across the peripheral portions of the bolt's inferior surface medially and laterally. Thus the maximum surface stresses are in the two transitional regions where component-bolt contact is altered from femoral-bolt contact to tibial-bolt contact. These areas of stress concentrations in the bolt are most likely to show wear. Such wear patterns demonstrating grooves toward the ends of the bolts have been clinically reported in removed hinge prostheses. The distribution of compressive stress within the bolt creates shear strains within the material which could lead to fatigue failure with repetitive cyclic loading. Such stresses can be reduced by

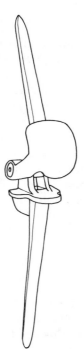

Figure 5.33. Hinged knee replacement prosthesis which allows only flexion-extension.

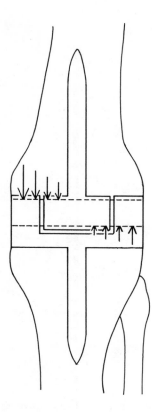

Figure 5.34. The bolt in a hinge prosthesis, because of the varus strain on the knee in gait, is subjected to compressive stresses as shown. The stress laterally is less than the stress medially due to the sparing effect from the addition of bending to compression (see Fig. 2.57).

designing the hinge so that contact of both components to the bolt is along the entire length of the hinge, and by increasing the diameter of the bolt.

The effect of the forces developed on the remainder of the prosthetic system (shank, cement, bone) as one moves away from the hinge follow the same principles as does the femoral shank in total hip replacements. About the knee the predominant forces are parallel to the prosthesis shanks and the long axis of the femur and tibia. Bending stresses in the prosthesis shanks are thus minimal and in the case of metal shanks there is little chance of these components breaking in these areas. Force from prosthesis to bony shaft is transmitted primarily with the development of shear between the cement and bone in a direction parallel to the long axis of the bone. These shear stresses can be alleviated if some force can be transferred by direct contact between the hinge and the distal end of the femur and proximal end of the tibia. This situation is similar to that of the hip replacement femoral component (Fig. 5.25).

If cement is interposed between the prosthetic collar and bone, failure is more likely to occur by either cement fracture or bone resorption at the contact points near the hinge's axis due to excessive compressive stress or by fracture at the bone-cement interface along the side of the shaft due to shear stress. The analogy to the hip replacement femoral component situation is clear (Fig. 5.26).

The more likely cause of loosening following insertion of such prostheses is torsion. The entire lower extremity is subjected to torsional forces in gait (Fig. 5.35). The rotational ristrictions placed on the system by the hinge create tor-

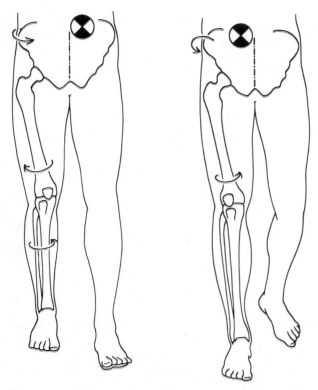

Figure 5.35. The lower extremity is always subjected to a torque in gait because we pivot over the stance leg. Normally knee rotation acts to diminish that torque.

sional forces and subsequent shear stresses in a plane perpendicular to the femoral shaft or tibial shaft. Since the hinge prevents internal and external rotation, significant shear stresses are created between the prosthetic shank and surrounding cement and trabecular bone. When such shear forces develop at the interface, the stresses they create are higher than the shear stresses parallel to the shaft as the circumferential area is smaller than the longitudinal area in these prosthetic replacements. Under such circumstances the shear stresses are highest in this plane and totally transmitted to the bone-cement interface.

12. SEMI-CONSTRAINED TOTAL KNEE PROSTHESES

In an attempt to maintain some nonligamentous constraint yet allow the knee replacement prosthesis to rotate in several planes to reduce the torques on the bone-cement interface, semi-constrained prostheses were developed.

The need for a knee replacement that does not depend on the cruciate ligaments for stability but provides adequate freedom of rotation could not adequately be fulfilled by the simple hinge prosthesis and spawned a multiplicity of "semi-constrained" designs. The first were captured balls (Fig. 5.36) added onto a hinge, allowing flexion-extension and rotation. They did not permit

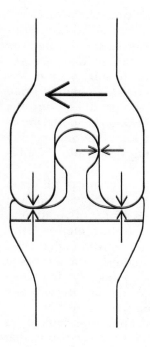

Figure 5.36. Semi-constrained knee replacement utilizing the captured ball design with added tibial troughs.

varus-valgus motion and were subject to fatigue failure, from lateral bending, at the base of the pedestal the ball sat on. Further, the necessity for condyles meant the ball had to be relatively small, creating significant stress concentrations in its polyethylene sockets, leading to polyethylene wear.

Subsequent designs have tried tibial troughs to capture the femoral component in the A-P direction.

Attempts to capture the femoral component by various lips and flanges on the polyethylene tibial component, peripherally and in the intercondylar notch, create stress concentrations which can easily push the polyethylene beyond its elastic limit (see Fig. 5.29 and Chapter 2, Section 4). This can cause cold (viscous) flow, wear, and eventual loss of stability (Fig. 5.37).

The amount of polyethylene that can be used is limited by the external size of the tibial plateaus being replaced and by the need to maintain large tibio-femoral

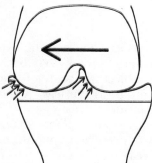

Figure 5.37. High stress concentrations on the polyethylene tibial component can be associated with its significant deformation.

contact areas to minimize the compressive stress at the articular surfaces. Large and broad tibial polyethylene lips to maintain stability concentrate the compressive, bending, and shear stresses and cause them to be transmitted through the prosthesis to the bone-cement interface. The distribution of these forces across a tibial cross-section is not uniform and the prosthesis tends to sink or tip downward in an area where compressive forces are concentrated. Depending upon the preoperative condition of the patient, the design of the prosthesis, and the surgical placement of the component, this tipping may be anterior-posterior or medial-lateral. In essence all such motion may be viewed as rotational motion which can be reduced by adding small shanks extending down into the tibia itself.

The effect of such shanks is much like the cement-filled holes one produces in the acetabulum during total hip replacement which increases the overall area of contact. It also places the area of contact as far from the center of rotation as possible and sufficiently increases the moment arms to produce high resistive torques to resist rotation with minimum forces at the interface. Although the use of pegs on the underside of the polyethylene tibial components of the knee joint prosthesis does improve the situation, to date it has not completely eliminated the problem. A trade-off continually exists between providing stability with motion at the knee while still minimizing failure at the bone-cement interface.

The more complicated mechanical demands of total knee replacement, as compared to total hip replacement, suggest a rational basis for predicting that successful total knee replacement cannot be based on a direct application of the designs used in total hip replacement. Clinical experience to date bears this out. Similar situations exist, with regard to replacement of other major appendicular joints, in particular the shoulder, elbow, wrist, and ankle. Designs for replacement of almost every other appendical joint have been made available to the orthopedic community, with mixed results.

Successful total joint replacement requires a complete understanding of the biomechanics of the joint being considered, an analysis of the nature and magnitude of the stresses that are created by joint replacement, and exploration of new prosthetic materials and methods of skeletal fixation. We have limited our discussion of total joint replacement to the hip and knee because we believe they clearly point out the general principles involved, especially the principle that each attempt at design of a different joint replacement requires different solutions for each joint.

13. POLYETHYLENE WEAR

In our discussions of the motions and forces at the interfaces between the two prosthetic components, breakdown of the surface material—wear—has been mentioned several times. Discussion of this important subject has been left for last because it is relatively the least understood and to date is the least noted clinical problem in the mechanical failure of joint replacement prostheses.

Wear is basically the removal of material from the surface. An implant can fail because of this owing to significant changes of geometry and, more commonly, to biological reaction to the wear debris. Polyethylene wear debris can produce

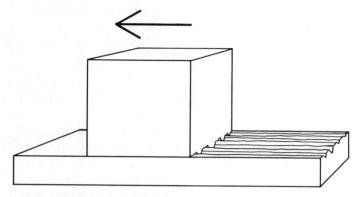

Figure 5.38. Abrasive wear. One surface scratches the other.

biological reactions which in themselves create failure. This has led to some failures in several knee prostheses.

There are three basic mechanisms of wear. The first, an abrasive type, occurs when an irregularity of one material, when moved over the surface of the other, scrapes out a path something like a plow going through a dirt field (Fig. 5.38).

The second mechanism of wear is adhesive wear. This occurs when the irregularity of one surface comes in contact with that of the other and because of simultaneous compression a chemical reaction causes one surface to adhere to the other (Fig. 5.39). Continued motion, however, must then break the two joint

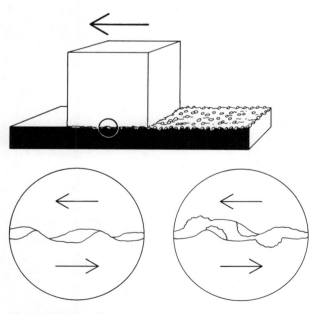

Figure 5.39. Adhesive wear. The tops of asperities adhere and are broken off at their bases.

materials apart and it does so at a different interface than when it was originally joined. The high spot so created on one surface is then prone to fracture. This may be likened to the ease with which stalactites can be broken off in ice caves or on the sides of houses in winter.

The third type of wear may also be considered an abrasive or adhesive type but of the third-body variety. Here, instead of the other surface ploughing through or connecting to the opposite surface, an additional material introduced between the two surfaces operates in the same fashion (Fig. 5.40). This may occur in total joint replacements from either materials such as HDPE rubbed off certain surfaces and remaining in the joint between the two surfaces or methyl methacrylate which may become chipped off from its original position or may have been loose in the joint since the time of surgery. In joints that have their surface contours so shaped that concave areas are facing downward, gravity may draw the wear debris into the joint rather than remove it, and are more susceptible to this type of wear than joint surfaces that are in the opposite direction. Example here could be cited of the difference between the hip joint and the knee joint.

The fourth type of wear that can occur results from nonuniformity of stresses at the surface, creating high compressive loads in certain areas and tensile loads at areas directly adjacent to it. The areas between them are therefore subjected to high strain, which if sufficiently large can create fractures. Because of the constant motion of the joint, this stress concentration is changing over a certain small area and if many small fractures thus occurring connect up, a piece of material may separate from its prosthetic source (Fig. 5.41).

Regardless of type of wear pattern, all are dependent upon the stresses which

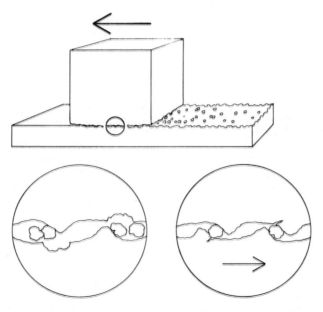

Figure 5.40. Third-body wear: debris between the bearing surfaces acts as an abrasive.

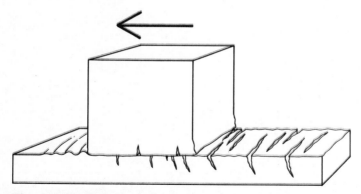

Figure 5.41. Fatigue cracks due to repeated surface stress.

are present in relation to the strength of the materials existing. In general, stresses in the knee joint are much higher than those in the hip, as contact areas are smaller. With regard to material strength, the hardness of the material is a good parameter by which to judge the degree of wear. If two surfaces are of different strength or hardness, wear occurs in the softer of the two. This may be altered if there is a certain chemical affinity between the two surfaces as wear may be accelerated by adhesive mechanism in this case.

The harder the contact surface, the less the wear. Less wear material is present on a theoretical basis if there is a metal-on-metal prosthesis than if there is a metal against high density polyethylene prosthesis. If, however, the material is so soft that it deforms and the stresses created are absorbed by this deformation, no true wear occurs, only changes in surface geometry. Such is the case in cold flow.

If an interface is provided between two surfaces so that the the two do not touch during movement, wear can be reduced regardless of what surfaces exist. This subject—lubrication mechanics—is discussed to some extent in Chapter 2 and mentioned in the beginning of this chapter. In total joint replacements albumin appears to stick to the surface of the metal, creating a boundary material keeping the two surfaces apart. It therefore acts as a "boundary lubricant." The exact nature by which the hardness of materials, lubrication mechanisms, and deformation of materials all interact to accelerate or decelerate wear varies greatly from material to material and is the subject of intense interest in engineering circles. At the moment for our concerns, we are aware of such conditions and with the materials available no major problems except for debris have been noted.

Attempts to make HDPE ultra high molecular weight or to impregnate it with other materials have given no proof that the resultant material has the overall wear properties of HDPE, and thus it is possible that improving one parameter of material structure may decrease some of its other ones. Only time will tell whether this is the case and if it is important or not.

Appendix: Explanation of Units

There is general movement toward a unified international system of units. Most scientific journals have adopted this "International System of Units" (officially abbreviated "SI") and require that British units and mks units (meter-kilogram-second, which is a subsystem of the SI system) be converted to the official SI units for publication. The SI system is based on six basic units, five of which are relevant to bio-engineering type of activity. These units are: length . . . meter (m); mass . . . kilogram (kg); time . . . seconds (s); temperature . . . Kelvin degree (°K); electric current . . . ampere (A). All other SI units are derived from these. Below is a list of the most important units (official SI units are italicized) and conversion factors for other systems.

Length: *1 meter (m)* = 100 centimeters (cm); 1 foot (ft) = 0.3048 mi 1 micron = $10x^2$ m; 1 angstrom = $0.1 \times 10x^9$ m; 1 inch (in) = $2.54 \times 10x^2$ m.

Linear velocity: *meter/second (m/s);* 1 kilometer/hour = 0.2778 m/s: 1 mph = 0.447 m/s; 1 foot per minute (FPM) = $5.08 \times 10x^3$ m/s.

Mass: *kilogram (kg)* = 1000 grams (g); 1 pound-mass (lbm) = 0.4536 kg; 1 slug = 14.594 kg; 1 ounce (oz) = 0.02835 kg.

Force: *newton (N)* = 100,000 dynes; 1 pound-force (lbf) = 4.4482 N; 1 kilogram-force (kg) [do not use kilogram for force, it is a unit of mass] = 9.8067 N; 1 gram-force (g) [do not use grams for force, it is a unit of mass] = $9.8067 \times 10x^3$ N.

Pressure: *newton per square meter (N/m²);* 1 pound per square inch (psi) = 6894.8 N/m²; 1 normal atmosphere (760 torr) = 101,325 N/m²; 1 bar = 10^5 N/m²; 1 kilogram-force per cm² [do not use kg/cm²] = 98,066.5 N/m²; 1 mm of mercury = 133.32 N/m²; 1 lbf/ft² = 47,880 N/m².

Energy, work: *joule (J)* = 1 newton-meter (N-m) = 10^7 erg; 1 foot-pound (ft-lbf) = 1.3558 J; 1 British thermal unit (BTU) = 1054 J; 1 calorie (cal) [try not to use calorics] = 4.184 J.

Power: *1 watt (W)* = J/s; 1 foot-pound (ft-lb) = 1.3558 W; 1 horsepower (hp) = 745.7 W; 1 BTU/hr = 0.2931 W.

In this text we use the SI units, followed in parenthesis by the British unit equivalent.

Selected Readings

CHAPTER 1

Lumbosacral Mechanics:

Farfan, H..F.: *Mechanical Disorders of the Low Back,* Lea and Febiger, Philadelphia, 1973.

Mechanical Properties of Materials

Hayden, W., Moffatt, W.G., and Wulff, J.: *Structure and Properties of Materials,* vol. 3, Mechanical Behavior, John Wiley and Sons, New York, 1965.

Physiology of Joints:

Kapandji, I.A.: *The Physiology of the Joints,* vol. 3, Churchill Livingstone, Edinburgh, 1974.

Biomechanics of Bone:

Kummer, B.: Biomechanics of Bone in *Biomechanics, Its Foundations and Objectives,* pg. 237, ed. Fung, Y.C., Pennone, N., and Anliker, M., Prentice-Hall, Englewood, N.J., 1972.

Spinal Bracing:

Atlas for Orthotics, Biomechanical Principles in Application, American Academy of Orthopaedic Surgeons, C.V. Mosby, St. Louis, 1975.

Mechanics of Scoliosis:

Riseborough, E.J.: *Scoliosis and Other Deformities of the Axial Skeleton,* Little Brown, Boston, 1975.

CHAPTER 2

Fracture Healing:

Pauwels, F.: *Gesammelte Abhandlungen Zur Funktionellen Anatomie Des Bewegungsapparates,* Springer-Verlag, 1975 (unfortunately in German but expect Springer-Verlag to publish an English translation within the next year or two).

Klenerman, L.: Experimental fracture in the adult humerus, *Med. and Biological Engng.* 7:357, 1969.

Lanyon, L.E. and Smith, R.N.: Bone strain in the tibia during normal quadripedal locomotion. *Acta Orthop. Scand.* 41:238, 1970.

Soto-Hall, R. and McCloy, N.P.: Cause of treatment of angulation of femoral intra-medullary nails. *Clin. Orthop.* 2:66, 1953.

Lawrence, M., Freeman, M.A.R. and Swanson, S.A.V.: Engineering considerations in the internal fixation of fractures of the tibial shaft. *J. Bone Joint Surg.* 51B:754, 1969.

Fracture Mechanics:

Klenerman: op. cit.

Hayden, et al.: op. cit.

Mechanics of Internal Fixation of Fractures:

Bechtol, C.O.: Engineering Principles Applied to Orthopedic Surgery, in AAOS Instructional Course Lectures, vol. IX, J.W. Edwards, Ann Arbor, 1952, p. 257.

Askew, M.J., Mow, V.C., Wirth, C.R., and Campbell, C.J. Analysis of the intra-osseous stress field due to compression plating. *J. Biomech.* 8:203, 1975.

Soto-Hall, R. and McCloy: op. cit.

Allen, W.C., Piotrowski, G., Burstein, A.H., and Frankel, V.H.: Biomechanical principles in intramedullary fixation. *Clin. Ortho.* 60:613, 1968.

Tonino, A.J., Davidson, C.L., Klopper, P.J. and Lincau, L.A.: Production from stress and bone and its effects. *J. Bone Joint Surg.* 58B:107, 1976.

Lanyon and Smith: op. cit.

Woo, S.L.Y., Akeson, W.H., Coutts, R.D., Rutherford, L., Doty, D., Gemmott, G.F. and Amiel, D.: A comparison of cortical bone atrophy secondary to fixation with plates with large differences in bending stiffness. *J. Bone Joint Surg.* 58A:190, 1976.

Lawrence, Freeman and Swanson: op. cit.

Mechanical Stimulation of Fracture Healing:

Latta, L., Sarmiento, A., Zilioli, A., Sinclair, W.: The role of soft tissue in the stabilization of tibial fracture. *Clin. Ortho.* 105:115, 1974.

Also See Clinical Orthopaedics Symposium on Practical Biomechanics which will be published in the next year or two.

CHAPTER 3

Gait:

Dec, J.B., Saunders, M.B., Inman, Verne T., Eberhart, Howard D., The major determinants in normal and pathological gait, *J. Bone Joint Surg.* 35A:543, 1953.

Inman, Verne T.: Functional aspects of the abductor muscles of the hip, *J. Bone Joint Surg.* 29:607, 1947.

Energy and Gait:

Elftman, Herbert: Biomechanics of muscle, *J. Bone Joint Surg.* 48A: 363, 1966.

Perry, Jacquelin: The mechanics of walking, *Physical Therapy* 47:778, 1967.

Joint Loading:

Denham, R.S.: Hip mechanics, *J. Bone Joint Surg.* 41B:550, 1959.

Tennis Elbow:

Nirschl, Robert P.: Tennis elbow, *Ortho. Clin. in No. Amer.* 4:787, 1973.

CHAPTER 4

Joint Physiology:

Radin, E.L., Paul, I.L., Rose, R.M., Simon, S.R.: The mechanics of joints as it relates to their degeneration. *AAOS Symp. on Osteoarthritis,* C.V. Mosby, St. Louis, 1976.

Radin, E.L. and Paul, I.L.: A consolidated concept of joint lubrication. *J. Bone Joint Surg.* 54A:607, 1972.

Mechanical Factors in the Etiology of Osteoarthrosis:

Pauwels, F.: *Atlas of the Biomechanics of the Normal and Diseased Hip,* Springer-Verlag, 1976.

Maquet, Paul G.J.: *Biomechanics of the Knee,* Springer-Verlag, 1976.

Radin, E.L., Maquet, P., Parker, H.: Rationale and indications for the "hanging hip" procedure: A clinical and experimental study. *Clin. Orthop.* 112:221, 1975.

Enneking, W.F. and Singsen, E.T.: Pathologic changes in the idiopathic painful cup arthroplasty. *Clin. Orthop.* 101:236, 1974.

CHAPTER 5

Total Joint Prosthesis Behavior:

Simon, Sheldon R.; Paul, Igor L.; Rose, Robert M., Radin, Eric L.: "Stiction-friction" of total hip prostheses and its relationship to loosening. *J. Bone Joint Surg.* 57A:216, 1975.

Galante, J.O.: Stress analysis of the femoral stem and total hip prostheses. *J. Bone Joint Surg.* 58A:618, 1976.

Semlitch, M., Reaction of the articular cartilage to plastic in metallic wear debris, from Joint Endo Prostheses. *Sulzer Technical Review,* St. Gallen, vol. 2, 1975.

Functional Anatomy:

Maquet, P.: His book on the knee, op. cit.

Radin, E.L.: *Newtonian Physiology: The Mechanics of Human Activity:* Scientific American, New York (should be published within the next two years).

Kapinji: op. cit. vols. 1 and 2.

Index